Fundamental Aspects of Adult Nursing Procedures

Also available in the current 'Fundamental Aspects of Nursing' series:

Fundamental Aspects of Adult Nursing Procedures
by Penny Tremayne and Sam Parboteeah

Fundamental Aspects of Complementary Therapies and Health
by Nicky Genders

Fundamental Aspects of Gynaecology Nursing
by Sandra Johnson

Fundamental Aspects of Men's Health
by Morag Gray

Fundamental Aspects of Nursing the Acutely Ill Adult
by Pauleen Pratt

Fundamental Aspects of Adult Nursing Procedures

edited by
Penny Tremayne and Sam Parboteeah

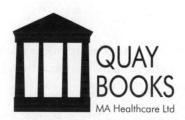

QUAY
BOOKS
MA Healthcare Ltd

Quay Books Division, MA Healthcare Limited, St Jude's Church, Dulwich Road, Herne Hill, London SE24 0PB

British Library Cataloguing-in-Publication Data
A catalogue record is available for this book

Printed in the UK by The Bath Press, Lower Bristol Road, Bath BA2 3BL

Contents

List of contributors

Mohamed Anwar is Senior Lecturer, De Montfort University, Faculty of Health and Life Sciences, School of Nursing and Midwifery, Leicester

Ricky Autar is Principal Lecturer, De Montfort University, Faculty of Health and Life Sciences, School of Nursing and Midwifery, Leicester

Anna Chesters is Senior Lecturer, De Montfort University, Faculty of Health and Life Sciences, School of Nursing and Midwifery, Leicester

Mandy Cooper is Advanced Professional Practice Cardiac Specialist Sister, University Hospitals of Leicester NHS Trust, Accident and Emergency Department, Leicester Royal Infirmary, Leicester

Mandy Gamble is Modern Matron, University Hospitals of Leicester NHS Trust, Leicester General Hospital, Leicester

Helen Gandhi is Freelance Clinical Nurse Specialist – Colorectal Stoma Care

Tracey Gray is Project Manager – Clinical Skills Development Unit, University Hospitals of Leicester NHS Trust, Clinical Skills Development Unit, Clinical Education Centre, Leicester Royal Infirmary, Leicester

Penny Harrison is Senior Lecturer, De Montfort University, Faculty of Health and Life Sciences, School of Nursing and Midwifery, Leicester

Graham Logie is Critical Care Outreach Charge Nurse, Anaesthetic Department, University Hospitals of Leicester

Barbara Marjoram is Award Leader, Academic Development Group Lead – Public Health and Health Promotion, School of Nursing and Midwifery, University of Southampton, Southampton

Usha Mehta is Ward Manager/Nurse Practitioner, University Hospitals of Leicester, Haematology Department, Leicester Royal Infirmary, Leicester

Helen Miller is Associate Director of Clinical Education, University Hospitals of Leicester NHS Trust, Glenfield Hospital, Trust Management Offices, Leicester

Abigail Moriarty is Senior Lecturer, De Montfort University, Faculty of Health and Life Sciences, School of Nursing and Midwifery, Leicester

Sarah Odams is Critical Care Outreach Sister, Anaesthetic Department, University Hospitals of Leicester NHS Trust

Sam Parboteeah is Senior Lecturer, De Montfort University, Faculty of Health and Life Sciences, School of Nursing and Midwifery, Leicester

Pauleen Pratt is Consultant Nurse Critical Care, University Hospitals of Leicester, Anaesthetic Department, Leicester General Hospital, Leicester

Ruth Rojahn is Senior Lecturer, De Montfort University, Faculty of Health and Life Sciences, School of Nursing and Midwifery, Leicester

Ivy Rushby is Respiratory Nurse Specialist, Department of Respiratory Medicine, University Hospitals of Leicester NHS Trust, Glenfield Hospital, Leicester

Liz Shears is Senior Lecturer, De Montfort University, Faculty of Health and Life Sciences, School of Nursing and Midwifery, Leicester

Alison Shepherd was Lecturer, De Montfort University, Faculty of Health and Life Sciences, School of Nursing and Midwifery, Leicester

Carolyn Staley is Ward Sister, University Hospitals of Leicester NHS Trust, Accident and Emergency Department, Leicester Royal Infirmary, Leicester

Penny Tremayne is Senior Lecturer, De Montfort University, Faculty of Health and Life Sciences, School of Nursing and Midwifery, Leicester

Rose Webster is Lead for Education and Practice Development, Cardiorespiratory Directorate, University Hospitals of Leicester NHS Trust

Foreword

I was delighted to be asked to write a foreword to this book because it is one of the best texts I have ever seen on the subject.

It is essential when writing a book on nursing procedures to always be sensitive to the patient's needs. This book begins with those essential characteristics, which not only ensure safety and efficiency in delivering high-quality nursing actions, but also outlines the key factors of success, and the reasons behind them.

The reader will enjoy the way the information is presented and produced to encourage a reflective approach and a systematic style of evidence-based delivery. It is easy to follow and find the relevant procedures to each major system of the body. There is also a final miscellaneous chapter, which mops up any procedures and information that does not fit easily into the previous ones.

Within each chapter each procedure is characterized by a logical sequence of steps taking the reader through the reasons for the appropriate action, the pre- and post-preparation, the equipment needed and of course a clear outline of what to do during the procedure itself. All this data is supplemented by further essential information, which adds to the usefulness of the book in clinical practice.

The book is well referenced and based on good evidence for nursing practice, which should make it an essential contribution to the nursing literature.

I know that all nurses whatever their background will enjoy it and I am confident will use it as a reliable reference work.

The authors are to be congratulated on an excellent piece of work, which should be widely available and accessible in clinical areas. Even better still I would urge nurses to purchase a copy for themselves. Certainly they owe it to their patients and themselves to be up to date, confident and competent in what they are doing.

Professor George Castledine
November 2005

Chapter 1

Essential requirements for nursing procedures

This chapter identifies areas of practice that must be considered before any procedure can take place to ensure that patients receive quality care by competent professional nurses. The areas to be included are:

⌘ Consent to treatment
⌘ Dignity
⌘ Privacy
⌘ Comfort.

In addition, all procedures must be accompanied by accurate documentation to demonstrate that the duty of care has been fulfilled, to enable continuity of care and to show the nurse's professionalism. Part of the preparation for procedures must always be to ensure that health and safety, infection control and local and, if applicable, national policies and procedures are adhered to.

Consent to treatment

The NHS Plan (Department of Health (DoH), 2000) identified the need for changes in the way that patients are asked to give their consent, to ensure that the process becomes properly focused on the rights of individual patients. Consent is a unifying principle, representing the legal and ethical expression of the human right to have one's autonomy and self-determination respected (McHale et al, 1997).

The intention of consent is to protect and respect a patient's autonomy and to promote meaningful decision-making (Aveyard, 2001; Beauchamp and Childress, 2001; DoH, 2001a; Nursing and Midwifery Council (NMC), 2002; Cable et al, 2003; Dimond, 2003).

Obtaining consent is a fundamental part of good practice, and any healthcare professional who does not obtain valid consent may be liable to legal action by the patient, in either a civil or criminal offence of battery or in a claim for negligence. They would also find themselves having to account for their actions to the appropriate professional body (DoH, 2001a).

Before any procedure in this book is performed, the practitioner must possess knowledge and understanding of the subject of consent so that a valid and meaningful consent is obtained before continuing with the procedure.

Types of consent

Consent may be expressed explicitly or implied. It can be given verbally, in writing or implied by conduct, depending on the clinical situation, the treatment and the degree of risk involved.

Implied consent

Implied consent is a universally accepted concept; it relates to the behaviour of the patient that indicates to the healthcare professional his/her agreement to the procedure. Implied consent is often obtained for simple acts of care, such as mobilizing or personal hygiene.

Aveyard (2002) advises caution when relying on implied consent for nursing procedures because of the difficulty in distinguishing between consent and compliance. If any doubt exists, it is prudent to obtain express consent instead.

Express consent

Express consent is the umbrella term incorporating written and oral consent, used for procedures carrying a special risk. The law does not specify when consent should be written rather than oral (Kennedy and Grubb, 2000; Montgomery, 2003). Written consent is normally gained by the use of a consent form and draws the patient's attention to the fact that he/she is consenting to a clinical procedure, and that it may carry risks and have major consequences.

Dyer (1992) suggests that practitioners have a fixation on written consent and describes this as a triumph of myth over reality – it is the reality of consent that matters, not its form.

There is no legal, ethical or professional distinction to be drawn between the efficacy of written, oral and implied consent except in evidential terms. The crucial factor in all of these is the validity of the consent (Kennedy and Grubb, 2000; DoH, 2001a; Dimond, 2003; Montgomery, 2003).

Validity of consent

Gillon (1986) defines valid consent as:

> *'A voluntary and uncoerced decision made by a competent or autonomous person on the basis of adequate information and deliberation to accept or reject some proposed course of action that will affect them.'*

For consent to be valid, certain conditions must apply. The consent must be given voluntarily without coercion by a mentally competent individual who has been given adequate information (Kennedy and Grubb, 2000; Aveyard, 2001; DoH, 2001a; NMC, 2002; Montgomery, 2003).

Information

Information is a complex area and much debate exists over the amount of information that a patient needs. For consent to be legally valid, the patient needs to understand in broad terms the nature and purpose of the procedure (DoH, 2001a). Although this would avoid a claim for battery, to avoid a claim for negligence and sufficiently fulfil the duty of care to the patient, information should be tailored to his/her individual needs.

In relation to procedures in this book, the information given must demonstrate knowledge of the procedure, be individualized and given in an understandable format. Kennedy (2001) recommends that information should be given in a variety of ways, should be given in stages and should be reinforced over time. It should be tailored to the needs, circumstances and wishes of the individual; it should be based on current evidence, in a form that is comprehensible to patients.

When performing nursing procedures, information should be given on what the procedure is, why it is necessary, the perceived benefits and risks, the available alternatives and the consequences of not performing the procedure. The information should be presented in a way that can be easily understood, avoiding the use of jargon. The patient should be allowed time to ask questions and have them answered honestly. The information-giving process should be ongoing where possible throughout the procedure, and the conversations documented to establish that valid consent was obtained.

Each individual patient will require different amounts of information and there will be those who do not wish to receive information at all. In this case, their wishes must be respected and again the decision documented.

Voluntary

Consent must be voluntary, free from force, deceit, duress, overreaching or other ulterior forms of constraint. Such pressure can be evident from family members as well as healthcare professionals. Patients must know they can refuse care and ask questions (Alderson and Goodey, 1998).

Capacity

The NMC (2002) states that you should presume that every patient and client is legally competent unless otherwise assessed by a suitably qualified practitioner. Capacity is generally characterized by understanding. If a patient refuses a procedure, it does not mean that he/she lacks capacity, it might just be that he/she has a different opinion and set of values. In these instances, the nurse must ensure that the patient has received all the information needed to make a decision and that the refusal is documented.

If a patient lacks capacity to consent for the procedure, it may still go ahead if it is considered in the patient's best interest.

Care without consent

In emergencies where treatment is necessary to preserve life or where the capacity of the patient is permanent or likely to be long-standing, it is lawful to carry out procedures that are in the best interest of the patient (Kennedy and Grubb, 2000; DoH, 2001a; 2002; NMC, 2002; Cable et al, 2003; Dimond, 2003; Montgomery, 2003). Best interests are not confined to medical best interests but include the patient's values and preferences when competent. These include their:

⌘ Psychological health, wellbeing and quality of life
⌘ Relationships with family and other carers
⌘ Spiritual and religious welfare
⌘ Own financial interests (DoH, 2001a).

When a person lacks the capacity to consent, either permanently or temporarily, no other person in English or Welsh Law is able to consent on their behalf. Views of significant people are considered; however, the ultimate responsibility for acting in the patient's best interests is the clinician (Kennedy and Grubb, 2000; DoH, 2001a; Dimond, 2003; Montgomery, 2003).

Who should obtain consent?

Ideally, the individual performing the procedure should obtain consent. This is particularly appropriate for the procedures in this book, where oral consent is likely to be sought at the point when the procedure will be carried out. At other times, it may not be possible for the person carrying out the procedure to obtain the consent. In such circumstances, the task may be delegated to nurses on behalf of a colleague.

The NMC (2002) affirms that you may seek consent on behalf of colleagues if you have been specially trained for that area of practice.

The DoH (2002) acknowledges this practice as long as professionals are competent to do so, either because they are to carry out the procedure or because they have received specialist training in advising patients about the procedure, and they have been assessed, are aware of their own knowledge limitations and are subject to audit.

When should consent be sought?

The process of consent may take place at one time or over a series of meetings and discussions. The DoH (2002) describes this as single-stage consent and as a process of two or more stages. The latter is particularly pertinent to elective surgery or procedures and treatments where there is an initial decision and when later discussions confirm that the patient, after having had time to absorb the information and ensured understanding, still wants to go ahead.

Single-stage consent is the process for obtaining consent most likely for the procedures within this book, where the procedure is initiated immediately after the explanation and after ascertaining that the required competence and lack of coercion exist.

Withdrawal of consent during the procedure

A patient with capacity is entitled to withdraw consent at any time, including during the performance of a procedure. If this happens, it is good practice if safe to do so to stop the procedure and ascertain the concerns while also providing an explanation of the consequences of stopping. If it is deemed to be life threatening to stop the procedure, the individual carrying out the procedure may carry on until the imminent danger has passed.

This section has explored the issues that nurses need to be aware of for obtaining consent prior to any nursing procedure. It has highlighted that consent is primarily concerned with protecting patients' autonomy and placing them at the centre of the decision-making process. By adhering to these principles and supporting them with effective documentation, nurses are demonstrating their knowledge to patients and are also enhancing the quality of patients' experience. This can include enhancing their dignity, privacy and comfort — issues that will be discussed next.

Dignity

The concept of the maintenance of dignity is central to good nursing practice (Haddock, 1996; Walsh and Kowanko, 2002). Nurses are advised through the *Code of Professional Conduct* (NMC, 2002) that they are:

> '...*personally accountable for ensuring that they promote and protect the interests and dignity of patients and clients, irrespective of gender, age, race, ability, sexuality, economic status, lifestyle, cultural and religious or political beliefs.*'

In order to maintain patient dignity, it is necessary to treat the person inside the patient, not merely regard the patient as an object or a disease in a body in a bed. Woogara (2001) links the concept of dignity to Article 8 of the 1998 Human Rights Act, highlighting that individual patients should be treated as persons, and that the quality of care is improved by respecting their wishes and dignity. Jacelon (2003) suggests dignity is defined as an individual's self-worth, composed of individual and interpersonal attributes, and something that is both bestowed by others in the immediate environment and exists independently of it.

The *Essence of Care* (DoH, 2001b) identifies nine key areas of care that have been identified by patients as needing attention. Included in this are privacy and dignity, which are now firmly re-established at the forefront of nursing.

Walsh and Kowanko (2002) compared the perceptions of nurses and patients with regards to dignity. The emerging themes are identified in *Table 1.1*.

Table 1.1: Patients' and nurses' perceptions of dignity

Patients' perceptions of dignity	Not being exposed
	Having enough time
	Not being rushed
	Having time to decide
	Being seen as a person
	Not seeing the body as an object
	Being acknowledged
	Consideration
	Discretion
Nurses' perceptions of dignity	Privacy of the body
	Private space
	Consideration of emotions
	Giving time
	Viewing the patient as a person
	Not treating the body as an object
	Showing respect
	Giving control
	Advocacy

From Walsh and Kowanko (2002)

How to maintain dignity

All procedures in this book require that dignity is maintained as an essential component. This should be considered pre-, during and post-procedure.

Pre-procedure

The nurse should establish effective communication with the patient by simple actions such as introducing him/herself and establishing how the patient would like to be addressed. It must never be assumed that it is always appropriate or acceptable to greet a patient on first-name terms. Failure to recognize and observe this courtesy can often threaten dignity. At this point the nurse must ensure that the patient is informed about the procedure and that he/she is offered choice (see 'Consent to treatment').

Walsh and Kowanko (2002) identified that patients felt that their dignity had been maintained when they were given choice and control. Not only should the patient be fully prepared before the commencement of a procedure, but also the environment should by ensuring that all necessary equipment is ready and checked and that the practitioner is competent in its use and aware of any pertinent health and safety regulations, policies and procedures. This enables the procedure to advance without interruption. Dignity is enhanced by ensuring that the patient is made aware that he/she is the most important person at that moment in time.

During the procedure

Mairis (1994) suggested that one of the characteristics of dignity is appreciation of individual standards, which are given little consideration unless one becomes vulnerable or anticipates their loss. This is evident during nursing procedures, and emphasis should be given to maintaining personal standards. Patient dignity can be achieved by ensuring the patient's comfort (discussed below), maintaining communication, giving reassurance, ensuring that the patient's body is not unnecessarily exposed or violated and creating an environment that remains private throughout.

Post-procedure

Communication, once more, is of paramount importance in order to give consideration to the individual's emotions and to provide time for him/her to ask questions or to express how he/she is feeling. It is important to ensure that any clothing is replaced and that the patient's appearance is acceptable to him/her.

All interactions that take place need to be patient-focused and not for the benefit of the nurse. Haddock (1996) suggests that the most powerful tool a nurse possesses to maintain and promote dignity is his/her own self, to work with feelings and to use them constructively to understand patients by treating them as valid, worthy and important at a time when they are most vulnerable.

Privacy

Privacy is inextricably linked to the concept of dignity. The Caldicott Committee Report (DoH, 1997), professional guidelines (NMC, 2002), *Essence of Care* (DoH, 2001b) and incorporation of the 1998 European Convention of Human Rights within British Law, have all raised the profile and expectations of patients regarding non-violation of privacy by healthcare professionals. Woogara (2001) highlights that respecting privacy is manifested in a multitude of ways – the right to enjoy and control personal space and property, the right to confidentiality and the right to expect treatment with dignity.

Breaches of privacy can easily be avoided during nursing procedures by thorough preparation of the environment. The major area for concern within the realms of privacy is that of confidentiality. This can occur in a variety of situations, such as asking personal questions in front of other patients during bedside handover and ward rounds. It must be remembered that while drawing curtains around a patient can successfully protect a patient's personal space, these same curtains do not provide a substantial barrier to prevent verbal confidential information from being overheard.

Documentation forms an essential component of nursing practice by demonstrating that competent care has been delivered. Part of the professionalism surrounding documentation is to ensure that data protection issues have been addressed regarding the storage of documents to ensure that privacy is maintained.

In conjunction with the confidentiality of information, nurses must provide an environment that protects personal space and privacy. Woogara (2001) identified that violation of privacy occurred when curtains were not shut properly or when people walked through curtains when procedures were taking place, thereby leaving patients in a vulnerable state. This can be avoided by clipping curtains together or by using a 'do not disturb' notice. An ideal environment would be away from the ward area altogether.

By adopting this approach, the professional is not only respecting a patient's privacy and dignity, but is also demonstrating the ability to maintain patient comfort.

Comfort

Comfort is an integral part of nursing care and has been cited as a desired goal since the time of Florence Nightingale. Achieving a state of comfort for a patient can be seen as a measure of quality care (Wurzbach, 1996; Malinowski and Leeseberg Stamler, 2002; Robinson, 2002; Siefert, 2002). The literature suggests that comforted patients heal faster, cope better, require less analgesia, have shorter stays and are generally more satisfied with care (Walker, 2001; Kolcaba and Wilson, 2002).

Tutton and Seers (2003) suggest that the exact meaning of the term comfort is unclear. Definitions have included comfort as an outcome of nursing, a basic human need and a process for which no consensus of a definition exists (Malinowski and Leeseberg Stamler, 2002). What is apparent is that comfort is broad, complex and individualized.

Kolcaba (1992) provides a technical definition of comfort as:

> *'...the state of being strengthened by having needs for relief, ease and transcendence met in four contexts of experience (physical, psychospiritual, sociocultural and environmental).'*

A patient attains relief by having specific needs met, for example by alleviating a severe discomfort such as pain or nausea. Ease is enabling a state of calm or contentment, and transcendence is the state in which one rises above problems and pain when they cannot be eradicated or avoided. This is of relevance during procedures when often discomfort cannot be avoided (Kolcaba, 1992; Kolcaba and Wilson, 2002).

The four contexts — physical, psychospiritual, sociocultural and environmental — are dynamic in nature and individual depending on the person and procedure. They could include:

⌘ Physical comfort with obvious needs such as pain relief, which should be considered and discussed before procedures
⌘ Physical comfort also encompasses issues that patients are unaware of, such as maintenance of homeostasis
⌘ Psychospiritual comfort is not easily identifiable, but could include issues such as touch and communication
⌘ Sociocultural factors should include being culturally sensitive, giving reassurance and support.

These needs can be met by employing good communication skills, developing a therapeutic relationship with the patient and by planning the procedure carefully. This may include having to inform the patient that you may have to perpetrate discomfort temporarily in order to achieve a higher degree of comfort.

Environmental aspects of comfort include issues that have already been discussed in relation to privacy and dignity to safeguard confidentiality and personal space. They also include providing comfortable furniture, diminishing odours and maintaining a safe environment.

A later definition by Siefert (2002) reflects these values and defines comfort as:

> *'...a state and/or process that is individually defined, multidimensional and dynamic; it may be temporary or permanent and requires that one's needs be satisfied in the physical, psychological, social, spiritual and/or environmental domains within a specific context.'*

For nurses to achieve a state of comfort in patients, there must be an understanding of the symptoms of discomfort (Robinson, 2002). Suggested symptoms of discomfort include:

⌘ Fatigue
⌘ Loss of appetite
⌘ Being too hot or too cold
⌘ Pain
⌘ Bowel distress
⌘ Loss of bodily control
⌘ Vulnerability
⌘ Fear
⌘ Embarrassment
⌘ Stress
⌘ Depression.

These characteristics again emphasize that comfort is indeed a multidimensional concept. Consideration must be given to the patient's comfort needs pre-, during and post-procedure, acknowledging that the needs will change at each stage.

Siefert (2002) adds that for patients to achieve a state of comfort they must feel that their personal safety and security is assured. This can include feeling comfortable they are dependent on knowledgeable and competent caregivers who have access to appropriate facilities and technology to meet their needs.

This chapter has identified some key concepts that must be considered before commencing any procedure in this book. It has also identified the importance of following health and safety, infection control and local and national policies and procedures to ensure a safe environment is maintained. In addition, it has emphasized the importance of backing up every action with accurate documentation to demonstrate that the duty of care has been fulfilled, to enable continuity of care and to demonstrate the nurse's professionalism.

References

Alderson P, Goodey C (1998) Theories of consent. *Br Med J* **317:** 1313–15

Aveyard H (2001) The requirements for informed consent prior to nursing care procedures. *J Adv Nurs* **37:** 243–9

Aveyard H (2002) Implied consent prior to nursing care procedures. *J Adv Nurs* **39:** 201–7

Beauchamp TL, Childress JF (2001) *Principles of Biomedical Ethics*. 5th edn. Oxford University Press, Oxford

Cable S, Lumsdaine J, Semple M (2003) Informed consent. *Nurs Stand* **18**(12): 47–53

Department of Health (1997) *The Caldicott Committee: Report on the Review of Patient Identifiable Information*. DoH, London

Department of Health (2000) *The NHS Plan*. DoH, London

Department of Health (2001a) *Reference Guide to Informed Consent for Examination or Treatment*. DoH, London

Department of Health (2001b) *Essence of Care*. DoH, London

Department of Health (2002) *Model Policy for Consent to Examination or Treatment*. DoH, London

Dimond B (2003) *Legal Aspects of Consent*. Quay Books, Salisbury

Dyer C (1992) *Doctor, Patients and the Law*. Blackwell Science, London

Gillon R (1986) *Philosophical Medical Ethics*. Wiley, Chichester

Haddock J (1996) Towards further clarification of the concept 'dignity'. *J Adv Nurs* **24:** 924–31

Jacelon CS (2003) The dignity of elders in an acute care hospital. *Qual Health Res* **13**(4): 543–56

Kennedy I (2001) *Bristol Royal Infirmary Inquiry. Learning from Bristol: the Report of the Public Inquiry into Children's Heart Surgery at the Bristol Royal Infirmary 1984–1995*. Stationery Office, London

Kennedy I, Grubb A (2000) *Medical Law*. 3rd edn. Butterworths, London

Kolcaba K (1992) Holistic comfort: operationalizing the construct as a nurse sensitive outcome. *Adv Nurs Sci* **15**(1): 1–10

Kolcaba K, Wilson L (2002) Comfort care: a framework for perianesthesia nursing. *J Perianesth Nurs* **17**(2): 102–14

Mairis ED (1994) Concept clarification in professional practice: dignity. *J Adv Nurs* **19**: 947–53

Malinowski A, Leeseberg Stamler L (2002) Comfort: exploration of the concept in nursing. *J Adv Nurs* **39**: 599–609

McHale J, Fox M, Murphy J (1997) *Health Care Law Text and Materials*. Sweet and Maxwell, London

Montgomery J (2003) *Health Care Law*. 2nd edn. Oxford University Press, Oxford

Nursing and Midwifery Council (2002) *Code of Professional Conduct*. NMC, London

Robinson S (2002) Warmed blankets: an intervention to promote comfort for elderly hospitalized patients. *Geriatr Nurs* **23**: 321–3

Siefert ML (2002) Concept analysis of comfort. *Nurs Forum* **37**(4): 16–23

Tutton E, Seers K (2003) An exploration of the concept of comfort. *J Clin Nurs* **12**: 689–96

Walker AC (2001) Safety and comfort work of nurses glimpsed through patient narratives. *Int J Nurs Pract* **8**: 42–8

Walsh K, Kowanko I (2002) Nurses' and patients' perceptions of dignity. *Int J Nurs Pract* **8**: 143–5

Woogara J (2001) Human rights and patients' privacy in UK hospitals. *Nurs Ethics* **8**(3): 234–46

Wurzbach ME (1996) Comfort and nurses' moral choices *J Adv Nurs* **24**: 260–4

Further reading

Department of Health (1999) *Making a Difference*. DoH, London

Morse J (2000) On comfort and comforting. *Am J Nurs* **100**(9): 34–8

Chapter 2

Observations

Blood glucose monitoring

Blood glucose monitoring is used to measure the capillary blood glucose. The most common site to obtain a capillary blood glucose is on the outer side of a finger. However, other sites are also suitable, which can be considered to be less sensitive than fingers:

- Forearm
- Upper arm
- Thigh
- Base of thumb
- Fleshy part of the hand
- Calf.

Results derived from a glucometer can be regarded as a guide only. More reliable methods are available such as a laboratory glucose or a random venous plasma glucose, a fasting plasma glucose or a 2-hour plasma glucose concentration. Such investigations may be undertaken to facilitate the process of diagnosis (World Health Organization, 2000).

Reasons for the procedure

- To establish the control of blood glucose levels over a period of time, indicating whether an adjustment in treatment regimen is required (Burden, 2001)
- To monitor improvement or deterioration in an acutely ill patient whose readings may be incompatible with his or her 'norm'
- To confirm hypoglycaemia/hyperglycaemia (Hall, 1999).

Pre-procedure

Equipment required

- Glucometer that is calibrated as per manufacturer's guidelines
- Pair of disposable gloves

⌘ Disposable lancet

⌘ Lancing device to which disposable lancets can be attached

⌘ Reagent/test strip that has been stored appropriately and is within the expiry date (check also when the bottle of reagent/test strips had been opened, as the shelf life of an unopened bottle is different to that of an opened bottle)

⌘ Soap, warm water, gauze/patient wipe (if patient unable to wash his/her own hands)

⌘ Watch or clock with a second hand (dependent on need — many glucometers have the timing component incorporated within)

⌘ Record chart

⌘ Sharps bin.

Specific patient preparation required

⌘ Identify and prepare the site of puncture by ensuring that the skin is clean

⌘ Wash the patient's hands with warm water

⌘ If alcohol has been used to clean the skin it must be allowed to dry as there is the potential that it may interfere with the reagent/test strip or biosensor (Blake, 1999).

During the procedure

⌘ Put on gloves

⌘ Attach the disposable lancet to the lancing device

⌘ Unsheath the lancet

⌘ Prick the outer side of a finger (avoid squeezing the finger), rotate or turn the finger so that a drop of blood can be placed on the reagent/test pad

⌘ To ensure an accurate reading, the drop of blood should cover the test pad and should be undertaken as one action and not a series of 'smears'

⌘ Wipe excess blood from the reagent strip after the recommended time, place strip in the glucometer and note reading

⌘ Remove gloves.

Post-procedure

⌘ Dispose of lancet in the sharps bin and return glucometer

⌘ Record the reading

⌘ Inform medical staff if the reading is abnormal (*Box 2.1*)

⌘ Review treatment regimen

⌘ Ensure site has ceased bleeding

⌘ Sites should be rotated to avoided complications such as hardening of the skin, pain and infection.

Box 2.1: Normal capillary blood glucose recording for a patient with diabetes

Before a meal	4–7 mmol/l
After a meal	No higher than 10 mmol/l

Student skill laboratory activity

⌘ Assemble equipment to undertake a capillary blood glucose

⌘ Using a range of simulated solutions, practise using the glucometer

⌘ Discuss result findings and implications for management.

Blood pressure recording

Blood pressure (BP) is the force exerted by the blood on the blood vessel wall. The BP is at its highest when the ventricles contract – this is known as the systolic pressure. The BP is as its lowest when the ventricles relax – this is known as the diastolic pressure. The recording of BP is regarded as one of the vital signs in the management of patients. The initial recording should measure the BP in both arms as this can vary and sometimes be significantly different. If there is no notable difference, one arm should be identified as the 'recording' arm.

Reasons for the procedure

⌘ Establish a baseline recording
⌘ Monitor haemodynamic stability
⌘ Aid diagnosis
⌘ Evaluate the effectiveness of medication.

Pre-procedure

Equipment required

⌘ Mercury/semi-automated sphygmomanometer device
⌘ Adult blood pressure cuff as recommended (Williams et al, 2004) (*Table 2.1*)

Table 2.1: Blood pressure cuff recommended sizes

Indication	Bladder width and length (cm)	Arm circumference (cm)
Small adult	12 x 18	<23
Standard adult	12 x 26	<33
Large adult	12 x 40	<50
Adult thigh cuff	20 x 42	<53

⌘ Stethoscope with clean earpieces
⌘ Recording chart
⌘ Pillow(s) to support arm(s).

Specific patient preparation required

⌘ Seat the patient for at least 5 minutes before measuring BP
⌘ Avoid caffeine and smoking 30 minutes before procedure (Torrance and Semple, 1997)
⌘ Expose both arms so that the brachial artery can be palpated
⌘ The arm(s) should be slightly flexed and supported at the level of the heart.

During the procedure

Manual BP

⌘ Locate and palpate the brachial artery
⌘ Apply the cuff to the supported arm, ensuring that at least 80% of the arm is encircled approximately 2–3 cm above the antecubital fossa, ensuring that the centre of the cuff covers the brachial artery (Williams et al, 2004)
⌘ To identify if there is an auscultory gap, palpate the radial or brachial artery
⌘ Ensure that the sphygmomanometer scale is easily visible
⌘ Inflate the cuff until a pulse cannot be felt
⌘ Deflate the cuff and mentally note when the pulse reappears — this is the estimated systolic pressure
⌘ Place the stethoscope, ensuring full contact with the skin, over the brachial artery
⌘ Place earpieces of the stethoscope into your ears
⌘ Inflate the cuff to 30 mmHg over the estimated systolic pressure
⌘ Open the control valve so that the cuff can be deflated at a rate of 2–3 mm/s
⌘ Mentally note the initial beating sound (systolic). As the cuff continues to deflate note the final beating sound (diastolic), noting the recording to the nearest 2 mmHg (Williams et al, 2004)
⌘ Repeat on the other arm (if appropriate)
⌘ Repeat another two times
⌘ Replace clothing.

Semi-automated device

⌘ Apply the cuff to the supported arm, ensuring that at least 80% of the arm is encircled approximately 2–3 cm above the antecubital fossa, and that the centre of the cuff covers the brachial artery (Williams et al, 2004)

⌘ Attach cuff to device following the manufacturer's instructions

⌘ Switch on.

Post-procedure

⌘ Record the mean BP on chart noting arm, activity/condition (Williams et al, 2004)

⌘ Inform medical staff as appropriate, noting the normal range (*Table 2.2*)

⌘ Clean stethoscope earpieces.

Table 2.2: Classification of BP levels

Category	Systolic blood pressure (mmHg)	Diastolic blood pressure (mmHg)
Optimal BP	<120	<80
Normal BP	<130	<85
High–normal BP	130–139	85–89
Grade 1 hypertension (mild)	140–159	90–99
Grade 2 hypertension (moderate)	160–179	100–109
Grade 3 hypertension (severe)	≥180	≥110
Isolated systolic hypertension (Grade 1)	140–159	<90
Isolated systolic hypertension (Grade 2)	≥160	<90

From Williams et al (2004)

Student skill laboratory activity

⌘ Assemble the equipment required to undertake a BP recording

⌘ Practise recording the BP of a person standing, sitting and lying down

⌘ Record the BP recordings on a chart

⌘ Discuss factors that may influence BP.

Central venous pressure recording

Central venous pressure (CVP) measurements can provide invaluable information about the patient's cardiac and fluid status. CVP is also referred to as the filling pressure, and provides a simple method of assessing the adequacy of a patient's circulating blood volume and the contractile state of the myocardium.

Central venous catheters (CVCs) are placed in the superior vena cava, just above the right atrium (Todd, 1998). CVP is the pressure of blood within the superior vena cava entering the right atrium.

CVP is measured either in cmH_2O or mmHg, depending on the system in use. The normal CVP is 7–14 cmH_2O (5–10 mmHg) when measured in the mid-axilla position, and 0–7 cmH_2O (0–5 mmHg) when measured using the sternal angle (1 cmH_2O = 0.74 mmHg) (Henderson, 1997). The difference between measuring a CVP recording at the axilla and sternal angle is 5 cmH_2O.

CVP lines can be inserted into one of the following major veins of the body:

- Subclavian vein
- External jugular vein
- Internal jugular vein
- Cubital fossa.

The CVC is inserted by the doctor, and the role of the nurse is to support the patient and assist the doctor. Once the catheter is in place, a chest X-ray should be performed to check the catheter is in the correct position and to rule out any complications. Regular monitoring of the CVP is carried out by the nurse using the manometer or electronic devices.

Reasons for the procedure

- To measure the CVP and assess the adequacy of the patient's circulating volume
- To observe a fluid challenge when diagnosis is uncertain
- To administer drugs that may cause local tissue damage if given peripherally, such as dopamine
- To administer fluids/drugs rapidly
- To gain venous access in the collapsed patient
- To administer cytotoxic therapy.

Pre-procedure

Equipment required

- Minor operations pack
- Sterile paper towel x 1
- Iodine 1% in 70% alcohol

⌘ Disposable scalpel x 1
⌘ 10 ml 2% lidocaine
⌘ 10 ml syringe x 1
⌘ 20 ml syringe x 1
⌘ Subcutaneous needle(s)/intramuscular needle(s)
⌘ Central line: single/multiple lumen catheters
⌘ Surgical gowns as necessary
⌘ Suture set and suture(s)
⌘ Sterile surgical gloves
⌘ Three-way tap x 1
⌘ Catheter Luer cap x 1
⌘ Dressing (film)
⌘ Drip stand
⌘ Water manometer set with 500 ml normal saline
⌘ Spirit level.

Additional devices for electronic measurement

⌘ Pressure-monitoring equipment and transducer assembled as per manufacturer's recommendations
⌘ Pressure bag
⌘ Heparin flush as prescribed.

Specific patient preparation required

⌘ The patient should lie supine with the neck extended and turned away from the insertion side
⌘ Place both arms by the side
⌘ The head of the bed should be lowered to encourage venous engorgement and ease of puncture of the vein (Peters and Moore, 1999)
⌘ After insertion of the catheter, three-way stopcocks are used to connect the catheter ports to the infusion set(s).

During the procedure

Recording CVP using a manometer

⌘ Place patient in supine position or in the position that the last measurement was made
⌘ Ascertain the point from which readings are being taken. This point should be marked on the patient to ensure that the same point is used every time. Record in the notes/observation chart
⌘ Stop all infusions running through the manometer line and flush the intravenous line to ensure that it is patent
⌘ Position the manometer and set zero level using the spirit level (*Figure 2.1*)

⌘ Turn off the three-way tap to the patient and allow the manometer to fill slowly to a level higher than the previous reading but avoiding the water reaching the filter at the top of the manometer

⌘ Turn off the three-way tap to the intravenous fluid

⌘ The water column should fall rapidly. When the fluid level in the manometer ceases to drop and oscillates with the patient's respirations, this indicates the CVP reading

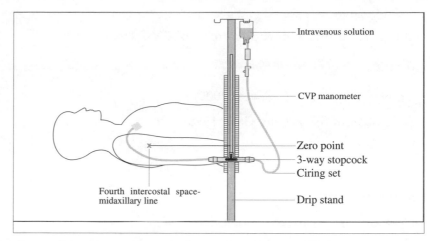

Figure 2.1: Measuring central venous pressure (CVP) with a water manometer

⌘ Turn off the three-way tap to the manometer and readjust the intravenous rate as prescribed

⌘ Make the patient comfortable

⌘ Record the CVP measurement on the relevant chart and report any changes to the nurse in charge/doctor.

Procedure for recording CVP using a transducer

⌘ The transducer should be calibrated as per manufacturer's recommendations

⌘ Position patient supine if there has been any repositioning

⌘ Monitor will display a CVP waveform

⌘ Measurements can be constant or intermittent, as required.

Post-procedure

⌘ The nurse needs to gain verbal and written confirmation from medical staff that the CVP line is correctly placed before using the line

⌘ Ensure all connections have Luer-Lok devices to prevent accidental disconnections

⌘ Use an aseptic technique when handling any connections

⌘ Change giving set as per local policy

⌘ Aseptically clean insertion site daily and apply transparent dressing

⌘ Inspect site for infection

⌘ Ensure patency of lines

⌘ Monitor for complications (*Box 2.2*).

Box 2.2: Potential complications of CVC insertion

Pneumothorax

Cardiac arrhythmias (Drewett, 2000)

Air embolism (Hudak and Gallo, 1998)

Infection

Arterial puncture

Catheter kinking

Haemorrhage – cardiac tamponade

Removal of the CVC

⌘ The CVC is removed when instructed to do so
⌘ Patient should lie flat with the foot of the bed elevated to prevent air embolism
⌘ Ascertain if the tip of the catheter should be sent to the microbiology laboratory
⌘ Switch all infusions off
⌘ Using an aseptic technique, remove sutures around the catheter
⌘ Advise the patient to take a deep breath in and hold
⌘ Remove the catheter by gentle pulling while applying pressure over the site with sterile gauze
⌘ Apply pressure for up to 5 minutes until bleeding stops
⌘ Apply an airtight dressing
⌘ Send specimen to laboratory, as requested.

Student skill laboratory activity

⌘ Assemble the equipment required to undertake a CVP recording

⌘ Practise recording a CVP using a manikin.

Measuring and recording respiratory rate

Respiratory rate is one of the most important observations that can be monitored and recorded.

One cycle of respiration is regarded as one inspiration (when air moves into the lungs) and one expiration (when air moves out of the lungs).

Reasons for the procedure

✳ To assess respiratory activity – the mechanics of breathing
✳ To facilitate more extensive assessment of respiratory function – the effectiveness of O_2 supply and removal of CO_2 can be ascertained
✳ To establish a baseline whereby improvement or deterioration can be determined
✳ For diagnostic purposes — the respiratory rate may be an indicator or sign of an underlying condition, such as heart failure
✳ To monitor for the effectiveness of treatment – to evaluate the efficacy of medical interventions
✳ To establish haemodynamic stability – to identify the effectiveness and functioning of body systems.

Pre-procedure

Equipment required

✳ Watch with a second hand
✳ Recording chart.

Specific patient preparation required

✳ The patient should not have undertaken any strenuous activity in the past 15 minutes
✳ The patient should be comfortable and relaxed.

During the procedure

✳ Nurses record the respiratory rate at the same time as they undertake the measurement of other vital signs
✳ Having counted the radial pulse rate, it is common practice to keep the finger in place and record the respiratory rate by observing the movement of the chest wall. Such a method can decrease the conspicuousness of the measurement of the patient's respiratory rate (Torrance and Elley, 1997a)
✳ An alternative is considered by Potter (2002), who suggests that the patient or nurse places his/her hand across the patient's abdomen or lower chest as this enables the respiration to be felt more easily
✳ If the rate is regular (*Box 2.3*), count for 30 seconds and multiply by two. If the rate is irregular, count for a full minute.

Box 2.3: Normal adult respiratory rates

Teenager	12–20 breaths per minute
Adult	12–18 breaths per minute

- Note the pattern of the respiratory rate (*Box 2.4*), and the depth of the respiration (shallow, normal or deep). This is regarded as the degree of chest wall movement.

Box 2.4: Patterns of breathing

Eupnoea	Quiet, normal breathing
Bradypnoea	Breathing is regular but slow, less than 12 breaths per minute
Tachypnoea	Breathing is regular but abnormally rapid, over 20 breaths per minute
Apnoea	Breaths cease for several seconds
Cheyne–Stokes respiration	Rate and depth of breaths is irregular, the cycle of respiration begins with shallow breaths that become increasingly rapid and deep, the breathing slows and becomes shallow again, only this time it is interspersed with periods of apnoea
Orthnopnoea	Difficulty in breathing when lying down
Dyspnoea	Difficult, laboured and uncomfortable breathing
Kussmaul's respiration	Deep, regular respiration, usually associated with metabolic acidosis
Biot's respiration	Breaths are abnormally shallow followed by periods of apnoea

From Torrance and Elley (1997b); Potter (2002)

- It is also important to observe and listen to the character of the respiratory effort — usually respiration is inaudible (*Box 2.5*)
- Record respiratory rate on appropriate chart according to local policy
- The respiratory rate in the elderly may increase, and this is primarily as a result of the decreased depth of respiration (Hogstel, 1994).

Box 2.5: Signs and symptoms of respiratory effort

Use of accessory muscles (the neck and shoulder)

Pursed lips

Nasal flaring

Sternal or rib retraction

Expiratory grunts

Coughing

Wheezing

Stridor (inspiratory crowing)

Stertor (gurgling, snoring sound as a result of tracheal or bronchial secretions)

From Torrance and Elley (1997b)

Post-procedure

⌘ Enter recording on appropriate chart
⌘ Leave the patient comfortable and reassured to minimize anxiety
⌘ Report abnormalities/deviations from the normal, so irregularities can be acted upon promptly
⌘ Amend nursing instructions as necessary so that other members of staff can clearly interpret what future interventions may be required
⌘ Consider factors that may have influenced the respiratory rate (*Box 2.6*).

Box 2.6: Factors influencing respiratory rate

Exercise

Anxiety

Acute pain

Smoking

Medication

Positioning

Neurological injury

Blood pressure

Student skill laboratory activity

⌘   Measure and record the respiratory rate of a colleague at rest and after climbing a flight of stairs.

Pulse oximetry

'Pulse oximetry measures the percentage of haemoglobin saturated with oxygen by passing specific wavelengths of light through the blood, usually via a finger or ear probe' (Fox, 2002).

Pulse oximetry contributes towards respiratory assessment but should not be used in isolation; rather it should be embraced within other assessment strategies.

Reasons for the procedure

⌘   Contributes to an overall respiratory assessment
⌘   Contributes to the indicators for further investigation such as arterial blood gas tension (pulse oximetry does not act as a replacement for arterial blood gas tension), but may also reduce the need for more invasive sampling
⌘   Facilitates the adjustment of invasive and non-invasive ventilator settings
⌘   Indicates the effectiveness of therapeutic oxygen
⌘   *'...assessment of tissue viability following vascular grafting or during the use of intra-arterial catheters. Any relative decline in oxyhaemoglobin saturation may indicate a decline in pulsatile flow and therefore a risk of developing limb ischaemia'* (Place, 2000).

Pre-procedure

Equipment required

⌘   Recording chart
⌘   Acetone (to remove nail varnish)
⌘   Cleaning equipment, such as alcohol wipe, soap, warm water, towel (to remove dirt and prepare probe site, especially if area is cold and clammy)
⌘   Working pulse oximeter that is charged if battery operated and has a safe mains supply
⌘   Appropriate probe for the site of recording
⌘   Clean probe.

Specific patient preparation required

✶ Remove dirt or nail varnish, as this can affect light absorption and the accuracy of the reading obtained (Jevon and Ewens, 2000a)

✶ Note the patient's condition — there may be factors where perfusion is poor and the pulse amplitude is small and may not be able to be recorded (*Box 2.7*), and readings may be inaccurate (Fox, 2002)

Box 2.7: Conditions/factors that may affect pulse oximetry readings

Peripheal vasoconstriction

Venous congestion

Motion

Dyshaemoglobins

Haemoglobinopathies

Bright light

Intravenous dyes

Nail varnish

Deeply pigmented

Optical shunting

Blood pressure

From Jevon and Ewens (2000b); Sheppard (2000); Fox (2002); Howell (2002a,b)

✶ Identify a suitable site to place the probe — this should have an adequate pulsating vascular bed (Jevon and Ewens, 2000b), and is usually a finger. Other sites can also be used (the ear or toe), but these are less accurate (Jevon and Ewens, 2000b). Also ensure the correct size of the probe.

During the procedure

✶ Follow manufacturer's guidelines for setting up equipment

✶ Attach the probe to the appropriate site, ensuring that the probe lead is attached to the oximeter and the pulse oximeter is switched on

⌘ Check the reading on the pulse oximeter. There may also be a waveform display that indicates the pulse quality at the point where oxyhaemoglobin saturation is being measured (Jevon and Ewens, 2000a). If pulse oximetry is continuous, note the site of the probe frequently and change position

⌘ If probe is in continuous use then beware of possible complications (*Box 2.8*).

Box 2.8. Complications of pulse oximetry and probe positioning

Blisters to the finger pad

Pressure damage to the skin or to the nail bed

Burns — patients with paralysis may have impaired sensation and therefore unable to convey discomfort

It is not advised that the probe is secured with tape unless the manufacturer indicates this. If it is secured too tightly it can inhibit venous pulsation

From Howell (2000b); Fox (2002); Allen (2004)

Post-procedure

⌘ Record reading on appropriate documentation

⌘ Undertake further respiratory assessments as necessary (observe colour, respiratory rate and rhythm, pulse rate, BP, chest movements, arterial blood gas tension)

⌘ Consider factors that may affect oximeter reading.

Student skill laboratory activity

⌘ Assemble the equipment to undertake a pulse oximetry recording

⌘ Record SpO_2 from the earlobe, fingertip and toe

⌘ Record the reading on a chart and discuss your findings.

Taking and recording radial pulse manually

The taking and recording of a radial pulse is a vital clinical procedure. Usually it is integrated within a number of other equally significant assessments that come under the umbrella of 'vital signs', such as temperature, respiration, blood pressure and oxygen saturation. McFerran (1998) describes a pulse as a series of pressure waves within an artery caused by contractions of the left ventricle. This can be further explained as the expansion of artery walls, in this instance the radial artery, when the heart contracts and pushes blood into the aorta.

Reasons for the procedure

⌘ Diagnostic purposes – the radial pulse may be a sign of an underlying condition such as atrial fibrillation
⌘ To monitor the effectiveness of treatment – to establish the efficacy of medical interventions
⌘ To establish haemodynamic status – to identify the effectiveness and functioning of body systems such as the cardiovascular, circulatory and respiratory systems
⌘ To identify change in condition – on admission a patient will have a baseline recording to establish their 'norm' at that time, so it can then be compared and contrasted with subsequent recordings.

Pre-procedure

Equipment required

⌘ Watch with a second hand
⌘ Pulse recording chart.

Specific patient preparation

⌘ Patient should have been at rest for a minimum of 5 minutes
⌘ Observe the patient
⌘ Identify suitable site for taking the pulse (*Figure 2.2*).

During the procedure

⌘ Place the first and second finger along the radial artery
⌘ Press gently with your second or third finger on the radial artery (*Figure 2.3*). Avoid using your thumb and forefinger as you may confuse the pulses in these fingers with the reading (Gale, 2000)

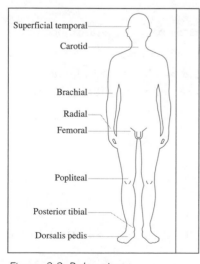

Figure 2.2: Pulse sites

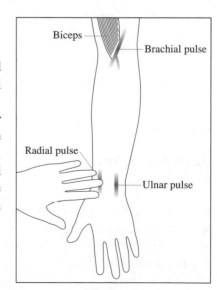

Figure 2.3: Radial pulse

❋ Count from zero the pulse rate for 15 seconds and multiply by four; for 30 seconds and multiply by two; or for a full 60 seconds (Hwu et al, 2000). It is suggested that the pulse should be measured for a minimum of 30 seconds, and if the pulse is irregular then it should be measured for a full minute

❋ Assess the heart rate (*Box 2.9*), rhythm, amplitude (strength) and equality (*Box 2.10*) (Torrance and Elley, 1997c; Gale, 2000).

Box 2.9: Normal and abnormal arterial pulse rates

Normal heart rate of an adult	60–100 beats per minute
Bradycardia	Below 60 beats per minute
Tachycardia	Above 100 beats per minute

Box 2.10: Pulse assessment, rhythm, amplitude and equality

Rhythm	Normally the pulse rhythm should have a regular interval. Interruption of such an interval by either early, late or missed is recognized as abnormal and can be labelled as an arrhythmia	
Amplitude	Usually the strength of the pulse rate remains the same. The pulse can be described as:	
	— absent, weak or thready	where the pulse is difficult to palpate and easily obliterated
	— normal	where the pulse is easily palpated and not easily obliterated
	— strong or bounding	where the pulse is easily palpated and cannot be obliterated (Torrance and Elley, 1997c)
Equality	Both sides of the peripheral vascular system should be checked to identify for possible obstruction, so radial pulses should be taken on the right and left side	

Post-procedure

❋ Record pulse rate on appropriate chart
❋ Leave the patient comfortable and reassured to minimize anxiety
❋ Consider medications, medical disorders and any other factors that may have an effect on the pulse rate (*Table 2.3*)

Table 2.3: Factors affecting pulse rate

Medications*	Medical disorders	Other factors
Anti-arrhythmics	Hyperthyroidism	Stress
Analgesics	Atrial fibrillation	Exercise
Beta-blockers	Cardiac arrest	Age (Hogstel, 1994)
Vasodilators	Shock (Armstrong, 2000)	Emotion
Muscle relaxants	Septicaemia	Pain (Fetzer, 1997)

*From the British Medical Association/Royal Pharmaceutical Society of Great Britain (2004)

⌘ Report abnormalities/deviations from the normal so that irregularities can be acted upon promptly
⌘ Amend nursing instructions as necessary so that other members of staff can clearly interpret what future interventions may be required.

Student skill laboratory activity

⌘ Identify the radial pulse and practise taking and recording this observation
⌘ Note the rate, rhythm, amplitude and equality
⌘ Discuss taking pulse from other sites as shown in *Figure 2.1*
⌘ Working in pairs, record how the pulse is affected by activities such as running, climbing a set of stairs and resting.

Temperature recording

Recording temperature is a valuable assessment tool in the management of patients. It is important that the procedure is performed accurately. Humans are classified as warm blooded and tend to maintain a core body temperature within fairly narrow limits of ± 0.5 °C between 35.6 °C and 36.2 °C, except when febrile illness develops (Marieb, 2004).

Body temperature can be measured in a number of common sites:

⌘ *Tympanic membrane.* The tympanic route is the preferred method in most hospitals. The temperature is measured by inserting a probe into the auditory canal
⌘ *Oral cavity.* Disposable chemical thermometers have mostly replaced mercury thermometers for oral use

⌘ *Rectal.* A rectal temperature can be measured by inserting a probe 3–4 cm into the anus. Rectal temperatures are generally 0.5°C higher than oral temperatures. This route is not commonly used because it is invasive, embarrassing, uncomfortable and unnecessary when changes in body temperature can be detected by other methods

⌘ *Axilla.* This route poorly reflects core body temperature because it is not in close proximity to major blood vessels. The site is more comfortable for patients and convenient for nurses.

Reasons for the procedure

⌘ To obtain baseline data so that changes can be detected
⌘ To assess suitability for treatment
⌘ To identify the presence of infection
⌘ To diagnose disorders of thermoregulatory function
⌘ During blood transfusion to detect transfusion reaction.

Pre-procedure

Equipment required

⌘ Appropriate thermometer (electronic, disposable)
⌘ Disposable probe (depending on equipment)
⌘ Gloves
⌘ Observation chart
⌘ Clinical waste bag.

Specific patient preparation required

⌘ Assess the patient regarding suitable sites for recording the temperature. If a site has already been used, this should be continued to maintain consistency
⌘ Ensure patient does not have an ear infection if using a tympanic thermometer.

During the procedure

Tympanic membrane temperature measurement

⌘ Follow manufacturer's instruction and familiarize yourself with the equipment before using the device

- Ensure lens is clean (if it requires cleaning, a dry wipe should be used; avoid using an alcohol-based wipe as it will lead to a false low reading)
- Insert a probe cover onto the thermometer
- Gently place the end of the probe in the external auditory meatus ensuring a snug fit (*Figure 2.4*). Advise the patient to keep his/her head still
- The thermometer should be held in place according to the manufacturer's recommendation (audible alarm/flashing light may be indicate that it is complete)
- Note the temperature displayed
- Dispose of the probe cover in a clinical waste bag.

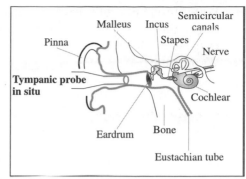

Figure 2.4: Tympanic membrane temperature measurement

Oral temperature using a disposable thermometer

- Follow manufacturer's instruction before using the equipment
- A patient's oral temperature should not be taken for at least 20 minutes if they have smoked, ingested food and drink or have been exposed to hot or cold temperatures
- Place the thermometer's sensor downwards (dot side) under the patient's tongue into either heat pocket as far back as possible (*Figure 2.5*). The patient should press his/her tongue down onto the thermometer and keep his/her mouth closed during this time
- Leave for 1 minute or as recommended by the manufacturer
- Remove thermometer and read immediately (following instructions)
- Discard after use.

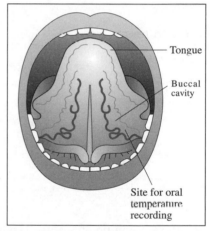

Figure 2.5: Site for oral temperature recording

Axilla temperature using a disposable thermometer

- Follow manufacturer's instruction before using the equipment
- Ensure axilla is clean and dry
- Place the thermometer in the axilla
- Place the patient's hand across stomach and leave as recommended by the manufacturer.

Rectal temperature measurement

- Patient lies on side with knees bent
- Insert probe in rectum and leave *in situ*
- Remove probe after recommended time

⌘ Wipe around patient's anus and make patient comfortable
⌘ Clean, disinfect equipment and dispose of equipment
⌘ Dispose of gloves
⌘ Wash hands.

Post-procedure care

⌘ Correlate results with patient history and signs and symptoms (*Table 2.4*)

Table 2.4: Signs and symptoms of pyrexia and hypothermia

Pyrexia	Hypothermia
Flushed	Cyanosed
Hot to touch	Cold to touch
Shivering/sweating	Shivering
Tachycardia	Bradycardia
	Apathy
	Drowsiness
	Poor judgment

⌘ Return equipment to its original place
⌘ Document the reading and report any abnormalities
⌘ Initiate care interventions as necessary.

Student skill laboratory activity

⌘ Gather a range of thermometers and consider their differences
⌘ With a colleague, record and compare an axilla, tympanic and oral temperature
⌘ Practise documenting the reading on an observation chart.

References

Allen K (2004) Principles and limitations of pulse oximetry in patient monitoring. *Nurs Times* **100**(41): 34–7

Armstrong DJ (2000) Shock. In: Alexander MF, Fawcett JN, Runciman PJ. *Nursing Practice Hospital and Home: The Adult.* Churchill Livingstone, Edinburgh

Blake J (1999) An insight into blood glucose testing. *Practice Nursing* **10**(19): 26–8

British Medical Association/Royal Pharmaceutical Society of Great Britain (2004) *British National Formulary 44.* BMA/RPSGB, London

Burden M (2001) Diabetes: blood glucose monitoring. *Nurs Times* **97**(8): 37–9

Drewett SR (2000) Complications of central venous catheters: nursing care. *Br J Nurs* **9:** 466–78

Fetzer SJ (1997) Professional nursing skills. In: Potter PA, Perry AG, eds. *Fundamentals of Nursing: Concepts, Process and Practice.* Mosby, St Louis

Fox N (2002) Pulse oximetry. *Nurs Times* **98**(40): 65

Gale N (2000) Observations. In: Mallett J, Dougherty L, eds. *The Royal Marsden Hospital Manual of Clinical Nursing Procedures.* 5th edn. Blackwell Science, Oxford

Hall G (1999) Blood glucose monitoring. *Practice Nurse* **18**(9): 618–20

Henderson N (1997) Central venous lines. *Nurs Stand* **11**(42): 49–54

Hogstel MO (1994) Vital signs are really vital in the old. *Geriatr Nurs* **15**(5): 252–5

Howell M (2002a) Pulse oximetry: an audit of nursing and medical staff understanding. *Br J Nurs* **11:** 191–7

Howell M (2002b) The correct use of pulse oximetry in measuring oxygen status. *Prof Nurse* **17:** 416–18

Hudak C, Gallo B (1998) *Critical Care Nursing: A Holistic Approach.* Philadelphia, Lippincott

Hwu YJ, Coates VE, Lin FY (2000) A study of the effectiveness of different measuring times and counting methods of human radial pulse rates. *J Clin Nurs* **9:** 146–52

Jevon P, Ewens B (2000a) Practical procedures for nurses: pulse oximetry – 2. *Nurs Times* **96**(27): 43–4

Jevon P, Ewens B (2000b) Practical procedures for nurses: pulse oximetry – 1. *Nurs Times* **96**(26): 43–4

Marieb EN (2004) *Human Anatomy and Physiology.* 6th edn. Pearson Benjamin Cummings, San Francisco

McFerran T (1998) *Minidictionary for Nurses.* Oxford University Press, Oxford

Peters JL, Moore R (1999) Central venous catheterization. In: Webb AJ, Shapiro MJ, Singer M, Suter PM, eds. *Oxford Textbook of Critical Care.* Oxford Medical Publications, Oxford

Place B (2000) Pulse oximetry: benefits and limitation. *Nurs Times* **96**(26): 42

Potter PA (2002) Unit IV. Vital signs and physical assessment. In: Perry A, Potter PA, eds. *Clinical Nursing Skills and Techniques.* 5th edn. Mosby, St Louis

Sheppard M (2000) Pulse oximetry: a case study. *Nurs Times* **96**(27): 42

Todd J (1998) Peripherally inserted central catheters and their use in IV therapy. *Br J Nurs* **8:** 140–8

Torrance C, Elley K (1997a) Respiration: technique and observation – 1. *Nurs Times* **93**(43): suppl 1–2

Torrance C, Elley K (1997b) Respiration: technique and observation – 2. *Nurs Times* **93**(44): suppl 1–2

Torrance C, Elley K (1997c) Practical procedures for nurses – assessing pulse 2. *Nurs Times* **93**(42): suppl 1–2

Torrance C, Semple M (1997) Blood pressure measurement: the patient. Part 2.2. Practical procedures for nurses. *Nurs Times* **93**(39): suppl 1–2

Williams B, Poulter NR, Brwon MJ et al (2004) *Guidelines for Management of Hypertension*. Report of the fourth working party of British Hypertension Society

World Health Organization (2000) *Definition, Diagnosis and Classification of Diabetes Mellitus and its Complications*. WHO, Geneva

Further reading

European Economic Council (EEC) *Medical Technologies and Devices*. Directive 93/42/EEC

Fulbrook P (1993) Core temperature measurement in adults: a literature review. *J Adv Nurs* **18**: 1451–60

Henderson N (1997) Central venous lines. *Nurs Stand* **11**(42): 49–54

Hudak CM, Gallo BM, Morton PG (1998) *Critical Care Nursing: A Holistic Approach*. 7th edn. Lippincott, New York

Kenward G, Hodgetts T, Castle N (2001) Time to put the R back in TPR. *Nurs Times* **97**(40): 32–3

Peters JL, Moore R (1999) Central venous catheterization. In: Webb AJ, Shapiro MJ, Singer M, Suter PM, eds. *Oxford Textbook of Critical Care*. Oxford Medical Publications, Oxford

Todd J (1998) Peripherally inserted central catheters and their use in IV therapy. *Br J Nurs* **8**: 140–8

Woodrow P (2002) Central venous catheters and central venous pressure. *Nurs Stand* **16**(2): 45–51

Useful website

Diabetes UK

www.diabetes.org.uk

Chapter 3

Administration of medications

Administration of medications is defined as giving medications to other individuals orally or by other routes. In order to comply with legislation, national and local protocols should be followed when administering medications. In the UK, the Nursing and Midwifery Council (NMC) (2004) recommends that the administration of medicines should be undertaken by people whose names are on the Council's Register. The NMC (2004) also specifies that nurses are accountable for their actions or omissions when administering drugs, and that practitioners involved in administering drugs should exercise professional judgment and the application of knowledge and skill in clinical practice.

The administration of medications should follow the five principles of safe practice as recommended by Parboteeah (2002):

⌘ The right medication
⌘ The right amount
⌘ The right patient
⌘ The right time
⌘ The right route.

Medicines can be administered by different routes (*Table 3.1*), and choosing the most appropriate route optimizes the effectiveness of the treatment (John and Stevenson, 1995).

Table 3.1: Common routes for drug administration

Route of administration		Length of time for drug to act
Oral	Given by mouth or via a nasogastric tube	30–90 minutes
Sublingual	Under the tongue	3–5 minutes
Injections	Intramuscular	10–20 minutes
Injections	Subcutaneous	15–30 minutes
Injections	Intradermal	Variable
Rectal	Inserting drug into the rectum	5–30 minutes
Vaginal	Inserting drug into the vagina	Variable
Topical	Placing on the skin or mucous membranes	Variable

Table 3.1 *continued*: **Common routes for drug administration**

Route of administration		Length of time for drug to act
Inhalation/ endotracheal	Via the respiratory tract	2–3 minutes
Optic	Into the eye	Variable
Aural	Into the ear	Variable
Nasal	Into the nose	Variable
Intravenous/ intra-arterial	Into a vein/artery	30–60 seconds

It is essential that the patient's identity is confirmed each and every time a drug is administered. Gloves should be worn as indicated, and hands washed before and after the procedure.

Reasons for the procedure

⌘ For treatment of disorders
⌘ Used prophylactically to prevent complications
⌘ For diagnostic purposes.

Before a drug is administered, it must be prescribed by a doctor or a nurse who is authorized to do so using the relevant drug chart and as per local policies.

The prescription should be written legibly and should include the following:

⌘ The name of the patient
⌘ The identification number
⌘ The date that the prescription was written and the signature of the prescriber
⌘ The medication and dosage, the route of administration, the time of administration and the duration of the treatment
⌘ Any relevant information that will enhance the effectiveness of the medication (some medications should be taken with, before or after food).

Oral medications

The oral route is the most common and convenient method of drug administration. Medicines administered via this route include preparations in solid or liquid form.

Pre-procedure

Equipment required

- Prescription chart — check that medication is due
- Select medications as prescribed and check for expiry date, discolouration, precipitation and contamination
- Medicine pot
- Spoon if necessary
- Drink of water/juice
- Tray
- Gloves, if necessary.

Specific patient preparation required

- Patient should be sat up to aid with the swallowing of the medication
- Instruct patient on how the oral medication has to be taken (enteric-coated tablets should be swallowed whole, medications for gastric conditions have to be chewed and some medications are placed sublingually).

During the procedure

- Check the labels and select the right medications in the right amounts
- Dispense medications using a non-touch method
- Empty the required dose into a medicine pot
- Take the medication(s) and the prescription chart to the patient
- Check and confirm the patient's identity and the drug to be given
- Give the medication to the patient in the medicine pot and a drink of water
- Instruct the patient to take the medication
- Ensure that the patient has taken the medication.

Post-procedure

⌘ Ask the patient to stay upright for a few minutes
⌘ Clear all equipment
⌘ Record in the prescription chart that the drug has been given
⌘ Complete all other documentation.

Administering medications via a nasogastric tube

Pre-procedure

Equipment required

⌘ Prescription chart — check that medication is due
⌘ Select medications as prescribed and check for expiry date, discolouration, precipitation and contamination
⌘ Medicine pot and adaptor to withdraw medications from a bottle if necessary
⌘ Prepare drug(s) following manufacturer's guidelines and advice from the pharmacist (James, 2004)
⌘ 50 ml syringe barrel
⌘ Tray
⌘ Gloves, if necessary
⌘ 50 ml sterile water to flush tube.

Specific patient preparation required

⌘ If the patient's condition permits, elevate his/her head 30–45° to avoid regurgitation and aspiration (Taylor, 1989; Pulling, 1992)
⌘ Following the insertion of a nasogastric tube and before the administration of medications commences, a chest X-ray should be performed and the position of the tube confirmed by a doctor before its use (consult your local policy as these may vary)
⌘ In an existing nasogastric tube, check the placement of the nasogastric tube by aspirating a small quantity of gastric contents and testing for pH (acid pH).

During the procedure

⌘ Flush the tube with 30 ml water
⌘ Administer the medication through a syringe barrel connected to the tubing

⌘ Hold the barrel of the syringe about 15 cm higher than the patient's nose and allow the fluid to flow into the stomach by gravity

⌘ Between medications and at the end of the procedure, flush the tube with 5 ml water

⌘ If the patient is on continuous feeding, the feeding is recommenced; otherwise, the tube is clamped.

Post-procedure

⌘ Dispose of equipment as per local policy

⌘ Document drugs given and sign prescription chart accordingly.

Drug administration via the sublingual route

Sublingual, meaning literally 'under the tongue', refers to a method of administering medications by placing tablets under the tongue or between the upper lip and gum. This route is recommended when rapid absorption and effect is required. The drug is absorbed via the blood vessels under the tongue, thus providing direct systemic effects.

Pre-procedure

Equipment required

⌘ Prescription chart

⌘ Medication

⌘ Small spoon.

Specific patient preparation required

⌘ Patient must be conscious and be able to follow instructions

⌘ Inform patient to place the medication in the buccal cavity and not to swallow or chew the medication

⌘ Patient should be informed that he/she cannot eat, drink or smoke until the tablet has been dissolved and absorbed

⌘ Inspect the oral mucosa for irritation caused by continuous buccal administration.

During the procedure

- Sit patient up unless contraindicated
- Check that the prescription is correct
- Dispense medication into a medicine pot
- Give medication to patient and ask him/her to place the tablet under the tongue/between the lip and gum
- Remind the patient to alternate drug placement sites.

Post-procedure

- Inform patient of the likely changes that may result from the administration of the drug
- Document medications that have been administered
- Monitor for effectiveness and complications.

Medications administered by injections

Nurses are routinely involved in giving injections intramuscularly, subcutaneously and intradermally. Therefore, only these three procedures will be described here.

Reasons for the procedure

- For patients who are unable to take medications orally
- If a patient is uncooperative
- When a more rapid effect is required
- To achieve high plasma levels for effective treatment
- If the medication would be destroyed if given orally.

Pre-procedure

Equipment required

- Prescription chart — check that medication is due
- Select medication as prescribed and check for expiry date, discolouration, precipitation and contamination

⌘ A clean tray
⌘ Select appropriate sterile syringe and needle (*Table 3.2*)

Table 3.2: Selection of needles for different injections

Type of injection	Syringe size	Needle size (adults)
Intramuscular	1–5 ml calibrated in 0.2 ml divisions	21 G x 1 1/4" (0.8 x 40 mm)
Subcutaneous	1 ml calibrated in 0.1 ml divisions	25/26 G x 5/8" (0.45 x 16 mm)
Intradermal	1 ml calibrated in 0.1 ml divisions	26 G x 3/8" (0.45 x 10 mm)

From Parboteeah (2002)

⌘ The length and gauge of the needle must be suitable for the injection site, the type of injection and injectate and the patient's condition. Volumes of <0.5 ml should be drawn in low-dose syringes to ensure accuracy (Zenk, 1993). For insulin administration, selecting the right needle length is important as insulin should be injected into subcutaneous fat rather than into the intradermal layer or muscle. As subcutaneous fat has a relatively poor blood supply, the absorption of insulin will occur over several hours and thus prevent hypoglycaemia
⌘ Alcohol swabs as necessary
⌘ Gloves
⌘ Sharps bin
⌘ Prepare medications if injectate is available in powder form or using a multi-dose vial as described in the subsequent sections.

Drawing medication from a single-dose ampoule

⌘ Check the ampoule for cracks, cloudiness and precipitation
⌘ Gently tap the upper area of the ampoule to release any medication trapped at the top of the ampoule
⌘ Use an 'ampoule breaker' to break the top of the ampoule
⌘ Insert the syringe and needle into the ampoule and withdraw the required amount, avoiding contaminating the medication
⌘ Change the needle and dispose of it as per hospital policy
⌘ Tap the barrel of the syringe to dislodge any air bubbles towards the needle and expel the air
⌘ The drug is now ready for administration.

Drawing medication from a multi-dose vial

⌘ Inspect the vial for cloudiness, precipitation and any damage

⌘ Remove the metal cover (initially) from the vial, clean the rubber cap with antiseptic solution and let it dry

⌘ Withdraw the prescribed amount of solution. Two methods can be used to draw the solution (Parboteeah, 2002):

— Insert a 19 G needle into the rubber cap to vent the vial. Insert the assembled needle and syringe, and draw up the required amount

— Assemble the needle and syringe and fill the syringe with the same volume of air as the medication that will be withdrawn. Insert the needle through the rubber stopper; holding the vial at an oblique angle inject the air into the vial. Keep the needle in the solution, invert the vial and allow the medication to enter the syringe. The volume can be adjusted by using the plunger. The needle is removed when the required amount has been drawn up

⌘ Change the needle as it may have become blunted/damaged

⌘ Gently tap the barrel of the syringe to dislodge any air bubbles and expel the air.

Reconstituting a powdered medication

⌘ Wear gloves as necessary

⌘ Clean the rubber cap with an antiseptic solution and allow it to dry by evaporation

⌘ Draw the required amount of water in the syringe as recommended by the manufacturer to maintain drug concentration

⌘ Insert the needle in the vial

⌘ Add the required amount of diluent carefully down the wall of the vial, and allow an equal amount of air to escape into the syringe

⌘ Remove the needle and syringe

⌘ Shake the vial gently to dissolve the powder

⌘ The reconstituted solution can now be withdrawn as described for removing solutions from a multi-dose vial.

Specific patient preparation required

⌘ Select an appropriate site for the injection. This is dependent on the volume and type of injectate to be given

⌘ Assess the site for muscle mass, blood supply, skin damage and for fibrosis as these will affect the rate of absorption of the drug

⌘ Consider a rotation programme if the patient is having regular and frequent injections, such as insulin

⌘ Consider alternative route if patient has a needle phobia.

Deltoid muscle

The deltoid muscle in the upper arm can be located in the lateral aspect of the upper arm. The injection site is located 2.5–5 cm below the lower edge of the acromion process (Craven and Hirnle, 1996) and above the deltoid groove (*Figure 3.1*). The needle is inserted at a 90° angle.

This site is used for small quantities (0.5–2 ml) of clear, non-irritating injectate. The patient can be seated, standing or lying down when this site is used for injection.

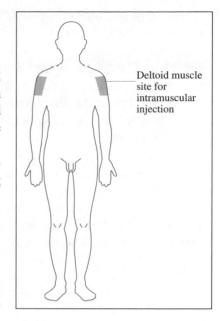

Deltoid muscle site for intramuscular injection

Figure 3.1: Deltoid muscle

Dorsogluteal site in the buttocks

This site is used for injections into the gluteus maximus muscle. This larger muscle mass is the preferred site for larger volumes (1–5 ml) of injectate. To identify this site, the buttock is divided into four equal quadrants by drawing imaginary lines to bisect it vertically and horizontally. The injection is placed into the upper outer quadrant about 5–7.5 cm below the iliac crest (*Figure 3.2*).

Another way of locating this site includes identifying the posterior superior iliac spine, the greater trochanter and drawing a line between these two sites. It is safe to inject above this line.

Bolander (1994) suggests that injections should not be given into this area when the patient is standing as the muscles are not relaxed.

Rettig and Southby (1982) recommend a prone or side-lying position, with the femur internally rotated to relax the gluteus maximus muscles.

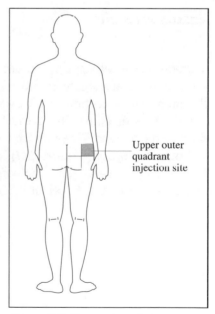

Upper outer quadrant injection site

Figure 3.2: Dorsogluteal site

Ventrogluteal site

Beyea and Nicoll (1996) recommend that the ventrogluteal site should be the primary site for intramuscular injections in adults as this site is relatively free of major nerves and blood vessels.

The intramuscular injection is given in the gluteus medius and gluteus minimus muscles. This site is located by placing the heel of the opposing hand on the greater trochanter (left hand for right hip). The index finger is then placed on the anterior superior iliac spine and the middle finger extended dorsally towards and below the iliac crest. The V formed by the index finger, the third finger and the crest of the ilium is the injection site (*Figure 3.3*).

Workman (1999) suggests that between 1–4 ml injectate can be given in this site. The patient is asked to lie on his/her side and bend the knee on the side in which the injection is to be given as this position helps relax the buttock muscles. Greenway (2004) suggests that the injection can be given in a seated position as long as the landmarks and injection site have been clearly identified.

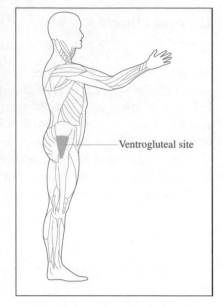

Figure 3.3: Ventrogluteal site

Vastus lateralis

This muscle is situated in the lateral thigh and is preferable to other sites because there are no major blood vessels or nerves in the area. The injection site can be identified by placing one hand's breadth below the greater trochanter at the top of the thigh and one hand's breadth from the knee. It is safe to inject in the middle portion (*Figure 3.4*), and up to 2 ml fluid can be injected. The patient should be lying down, but the injection can also be given with the patient in a seated position.

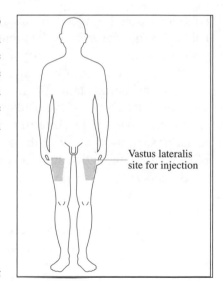

Figure 3.4: Vastus lateralis

Sites for subcutaneous injections/insulin

The most suitable sites for insulin injections are shown in *Figure 3.5*, with the abdominal wall and thigh areas being easily accessible for self-administration.

The injection site should be alternated between left and right sides on a weekly basis (Royal College of Nursing (RCN), 2004). The sites should be rotated within the anatomical site by giving the injection at least one finger's breadth away from the last one, as repeated injections in one site can cause fibrosis of the subcutaneous layer and may affect the absorption of the drug.

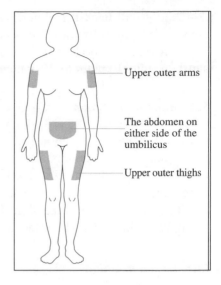

Upper outer arms

The abdomen on either side of the umbilicus

Upper outer thighs

Figure 3.5: Subcutaneous/insulin injection sites

During the procedure

⌘ Prepare the needle(s) and syringe(s) on a tray. Check for any defects
⌘ Check the patient's prescription and that the medication is due
⌘ Select the drug and verify it against the prescription
⌘ Prepare the medication as recommended by the manufacturer
⌘ Withdraw the appropriate amount of solution in relation to the prescribed dose
⌘ Check patient's identity band
⌘ Expose the site for injection
⌘ Follow local policies for cleansing the skin. If cleansing is required, the skin is cleansed with an alcohol swab and allowed to dry by evaporation. For subcutaneous insulin and heparin injections, alcohol swabs are contraindicated as they interfere with drug action and toughen the skin, making subsequent injections difficult (Burden, 2003)
⌘ Remove the sheath from the needle and place the sheath in the injection tray.

Intramuscular injection

For an intramuscular injection, using the non-dominant hand stretch the skin over the injection site. With the dominant hand introduce two-thirds of the needle at a 90° angle to the skin (*Figure 3.6*).

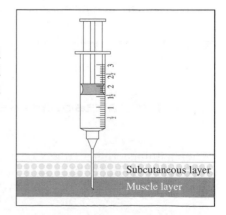

Subcutaneous layer

Muscle layer

Figure 3.6: Intramuscular injection angle

Gently pull back the plunger, and if no blood appears depress the plunger and inject the drug slowly. Quickly withdraw the needle, and if there is any bleeding apply gentle pressure over the puncture site. If blood appears in the syringe, withdraw the needle and repeat the procedure with a sterile needle. Explain to the patient what is happening.

Subcutaneous injection

For a subcutaneous injection such as insulin or heparin, the needle is inserted at 90°. Using the other hand, pinch up a large mound of skin and quickly push the entire length of the needle in at an angle of 90° and inject the medication. If using different systems and the needle is likely to go beyond the subcutaneous layer, pinch up a skinfold between thumb and forefinger and insert two-thirds of the needle at a 45° angle to the skin. The 8 mm needle is the length most commonly recommended for normal-weight adults who inject at a 90° angle into pinched-up skin (Wood et al, 2002).

Intradermal injection

For intradermal injection, select a lightly pigmented, thinly keratinized and relatively hairless area of the ventral forearm or upper chest, upper arm or shoulder blade (McConnell, 2000). Support the patient's arm and stretch the skin taut. Place the bevel of the needle almost flat against the patient's skin and insert the needle with the bevel side up at an angle of 10–15°. The needle should be about 3 mm below the skin surface, and up to 0.5 ml can be injected while watching for a wheal to develop. Once the wheal appears, withdraw the needle. The area should never be massaged as it may interfere with the test results. If the injection is for allergy testing, circle the injection site with a skin-marking pen for observation at a later date.

⌘ Place syringe on to injection tray. *Do not resheathe the needle*
⌘ Dispose of syringe and needle in the sharps bin at the point of use (RCN, 2000).

Post-procedure

⌘ Document procedure and report any abnormalities immediately
⌘ Dispose of equipment as per hospital policy
⌘ Document drug(s) given
⌘ Monitor for complications of injections, such as nerve damage, infection and muscle myopathy.

Z-track intramuscular injection

When administering an injection using the Z-track method, the skin is drawn away from the injection site (Belanger, 1985). As a result of this pull, the skin and subcutaneous tissues are moved away from the muscle, which remains static. When skin and subcutaneous tissue are released after the injection they return to their original position over the muscle. This return has the effect of breaking the needle track into the muscle because the track in the skin and subcutaneous layers move away from the muscle as the taut tissues return to the original position. This technique for intramuscular injection has been primarily reserved for use with medications such as iron preparation that are known to be particularly irritating and can permanently stain the subcutaneous tissue.

During the procedure

- The nurse administering the injection places the ulnar side of his/her non-dominant hand distal to the chosen injection site (ventrogluteal site commonly used)
- The skin is then pulled away laterally about 2.5 cm from the site and held taut
- The needle is inserted into the skin at the original site while the skin is still held taut, aspirated to check that a blood vessel has not been punctured and the medication injected slowly
- After waiting for 10 seconds, the needle is withdrawn quickly and the taut skin released.

Post-procedure

- Dispose of equipment as per hospital policy
- Document drug administered
- Be aware that this may cause elevated enzyme levels.

Transcutaneous/transdermal drug administration

Transcutaneous and transdermal drug interventions are non-invasive methods of administering drugs to the skin. The drugs are used for local effects or for systemic therapy. Medications for transdermal/transcutaneous use are available in liquid, ointment and patch form.

Pre-procedure – transcutaneous medications

Equipment required

- Medication as prescribed
- Prescription chart
- Gloves
- Disposal bag
- Gauze.

Specific patient preparation required

⌘ Some topical preparations may soil clothing. Additional clothing should be available
⌘ Skin may have to be washed with soap and water or special emollient
⌘ Do not apply medications to broken/irritated skin (McConnell, 2001).

During the procedure

⌘ Prepare medication for application following manufacturer's recommendations
⌘ Apply medication to the site as indicated
⌘ Avoid getting medications on your hands
⌘ Cover with appropriate dressings.

Post-procedure

⌘ Document drug administration
⌘ Warn patient of effects of medication
⌘ Dispose of equipment as per local policy
⌘ Monitor for irritation and sensitivities.

Pre-procedure – transdermal medications

Equipment required

⌘ Transdermal patch as prescribed
⌘ Disposal bag
⌘ Prescription chart.

Specific patient preparation required

⌘ Involve patient and ask where the patch should be applied as some patients may not want the patch to be left exposed.

During the procedure

⌘ Before any patch can be applied, the previous application is removed from the patient's skin
⌘ The new patch is removed from the packaging and checked

⌘ The new patch is then applied to a clean, non-hairy skin surface. The most frequently used sites are the chest wall, the upper arms, the backs of the hands and the antecubital fossae, depending on the intended use of the medication.

Post-procedure

⌘ Attach labels to the patch indicating the date and time of application and the signature of the practitioner
⌘ The site should be rotated and recorded on a rotation chart to prevent inflammation and irritation
⌘ If the patch has been properly applied, the patient is able to shower or bathe
⌘ Dispose of equipment as per local policy.

Eye medication

Medications used to treat eye disorders are available in liquid, gel or ointment form so that they can be applied easily to the eye without causing any damage to the delicate cornea. The gel and ointment formulations keep the drug in contact with the eye surface longer, whereas liquid eye drops may run off the eye too quickly and not be absorbed adequately to produce any beneficial effect. Ocular drugs are almost always used for their local effects.

Pre-procedure

Equipment required

⌘ Eye medication. Warm the eye drops to room temperature. Separate bottles for left and right eye
⌘ Prescription chart
⌘ Eye pads/dark glasses/eye protection as necessary
⌘ Adhesive tape
⌘ Eye toilet pack
⌘ Normal saline
⌘ Lint pieces as necessary.

Specific patient preparation required

⌘ Identify which eye is to be treated
⌘ If a fluid is being applied, inform the patient that he/she may feel some fluid is running into the nose as some fluid may drain via the punctum of the eye into the nasal cavity. The patient may also get a taste of the drug as it drains into the nasopharynx

⌘ Ideally, the patient should be lying flat with his/her head tilted backwards to allow easy access to the eyes. The nurse should stand behind the patient's head as it is easier to administer the drug from that position

⌘ Inform the patient of the length of action of the drug: anaesthetic drugs will have an immediate effect and may last for about 10 minutes; mydriatics and cycloplegics will become effective in 15–30 minutes and can last between 2–4 hours.

During the procedure

⌘ Remove any existing dressing
⌘ Examine eye
⌘ Clean eye as necessary
⌘ Open lid of the ointment
⌘ Gently pull down the lower lid to form a pouch
⌘ For the administration of eye drops, gently drop the required number of drops just inside the lower eyelid (interior fornix). Ask the patient to close the eye gently and blink several times. The nurse must wait for 2 minutes before instilling another drug
⌘ For the administration of eye ointment, start from the angle near the nose (the inner canthus) and work towards the ear, gently squeezing a 1 cm line of ointment along the inside of the lower eyelid. Avoid touching the eye with the sharp nozzle
⌘ An eye pad may be applied if requested. Separate tubes/bottles should always be used for the left and right eyes. The patient should be advised not to rub or squeeze the eye
⌘ Apply eye protection as required
⌘ Put lid back on the ointment container.

Post-procedure

⌘ Patient may have blurred vision at first and should therefore be helped to sit out
⌘ Some patients may prefer to stay in bed for a while
⌘ Document procedure and record assessment of the eye. Consider implication of eye drops when neurological observations are being recorded.

Administering ear drops

Pre-procedure

Equipment required

- Ear drops
- Dressing pack to clean and dry ear as necessary
- Prepare all the necessary equipment
- Shake the container
- Warm the medication to body temperature by holding the bottle between your hands for several minutes.

Specific patient preparation required

- Provide aural toilet as necessary to remove any discharges and dry ear canal
- Ask the patient to lie on his/her side with the affected ear facing upwards or to tip the head sideways.

During the procedure

- Open the container with caution and withdraw the required amount of medication
- Position the dropper tip near the ear canal opening
- Gently pull the pinna up and back to straighten the meatus
- Instil the prescribed number of drops into the ear canal. Place the drops onto the side of the ear canal and avoid dropping the medication directly down the ear canal
- Replace the cap on the container
- Ask the patient to remain in that position for 5 minutes
- Gently wipe away any excess medication
- Remove gloves and wash your hands
- Wait for 15 minutes and repeat the procedure for the other ear, if directed to do so.

Post-procedure

- Advise patient not to insert objects such as 'cotton buds' in the ear canal
- Inform patient that there may be some temporary hearing disturbance in the affected ear.

Nasal medications

Medications for administration via the nose are available in three forms: drops, nasal sprays/inhalers and nebulizers.

Pre-procedure

Equipment required

⌘ Medication as prescribed
⌘ Test nasal inhaler/spray to ensure that the system is working and also that there is sufficient drug in the container.

Specific patient preparation required

⌘ Ask patient to gently blow his/her nose to clear the nostrils and wipe any nasal secretions with a soft tissue
⌘ Ask the patient to keep head upright
⌘ Instruct patient how/when to sniff the medication
⌘ Patient may be allowed to self-administer the drug under supervision.

During the procedure

⌘ Ask patient to press a finger against the side of the nose to close one nostril
⌘ Ask patient to close mouth
⌘ Devices should be used according to manufacturer's instructions
⌘ Open container
⌘ Insert the tip of the spray or nasal inhaler into the open nostril
⌘ Ask patient to sniff in through the nostril while quickly and firmly squeezing the spray container or pressing the nasal inhaler
⌘ The patient is asked to hold his/her breath for a few seconds and then breathe out through the mouth
⌘ The procedure is then repeated in the other nostril as instructed.

Post-procedure

⌘ Monitor for effectiveness
⌘ Complete all records and documentation
⌘ Wipe away any nasal secretions.

Administering nasal drops

Specific preparation of the patient

- Instruct the patient to gently blow his/her nose to clear the nostrils and wipe any nasal secretions with a soft tissue
- Ask patient to lie down
- Inform patient that some of the medications may trickle down the nasopharynx.

During the procedure

- Ask the patient to lie on his/her back on a bed with the head tilted back and the neck supported
- Gently shake the nose drop container and withdraw the required amount of medication
- Insert the dropper tip about 0.5–1 cm into the nostril and administer the prescribed dose
- Repeat the above steps for the other nostril if prescribed.

Post-procedure

- Advise patient to stay in a lying position for 5 minutes
- Rinse the dropper tip with hot water and replace the cap on the container
- Complete all the relevant documentation
- Monitor for side-effects of bleeding or crusting
- Uncontrolled symptoms may occur as a result of poor compliance, poor nasal technique or incorrect diagnosis (Walker, 2003).

Medications administered by nebulizer

Administering a drug via a nebulizer produces a mist, enabling the drug to be inhaled directly into the lungs (Porter-Jones, 2000).

Pre-procedure

Equipment required

- Oxygen supply or compressed air box machine/cylinder
- Mouthpiece/mask

⌘ Nebulizer
⌘ Tubing
⌘ Drug/solution
⌘ Prescription chart
⌘ Peak flow meter.

Specific preparation of the patient

⌘ Sit the patient up to maximize lung expansion
⌘ Record peak flow if condition allows (bronchodilators are commonly given in nebulized form)
⌘ Forewarn the patient of the noise that a compressed air box machine may make to reduce anxiety
⌘ Establish preferred delivery device: mouthpiece or mask (the latter can make patients feel claustrophobic)
⌘ Encourage the patient to adopt a normal pattern of breathing when receiving the nebulizer.

During the procedure

⌘ Prepare medications as prescribed
⌘ Unscrew the nebulizer (in the middle) and pour the contents of the drug/solution into the nebuliser chamber
⌘ Screw the nebulizer back together
⌘ Attach the mouthpiece/mask to the nebulizer
⌘ Connect the tubing to the nebulizer and attach to either the oxygen supply or compressed air box/cylinder
⌘ Turn the flow rate on the oxygen/air cylinder to the required prescribed amount or switch on the compressed air box machine
⌘ Once the mist begins to appear at the mouthpiece, ask the patient to insert mouthpiece into their mouth or to put the mask on. If they are unable, place appropriately ensuring that the mask is secure.

Post-procedure

⌘ Observe for side-effects, such as tachycardia, tremor, palpitations
⌘ Offer mouthwash, as a nebulizer can dry the oral mucosa
⌘ Record peak flow to monitor the effectiveness of nebulized medication
⌘ Ensure that the nebulizer, oxygen mask and mouthpiece are washed at least once daily (Porter-Jones, 2000) or as according to local policy
⌘ Document in prescription chart.

Administration of medications via the rectal route

Medications for administration via the rectal route include enemas and suppositories:

- An enema is a quantity of fluid infused into the rectum through a tube passed into the anus
- Suppositories are solid, bullet-shaped preparations designed for easy insertion into the anus.

Rectal medications can be used to alleviate constipation, to clean the lower bowel and rectum before surgery, for therapeutic purposes and to prevent complications of nausea and vomiting often associated with the oral route (Shepherd, 2002). Rectal administration of medications is contraindicated in cases of abdominal pain, bowel obstruction, lower bowel surgery and infection.

Administration of an enema

Equipment required

- Disposable apron and gloves
- Disposable wipes/toilet tissues, soap and water/towels
- Disposable incontinence sheets to protect the bed
- Enema as prescribed
- Warm the enema in a jug of hot water to body temperature
- Water-soluble lubricant
- Ensure toileting facilities are ready.

Specific patient preparation required

- Ask patient to empty his/her bladder before the procedure
- Inform patient to retain the enema for as long as possible for maximum effectiveness and that bowel action thereafter may become volatile
- The patient should lie on the left side with knees flexed and the buttocks closer to the edge of the bed
- Place protective sheets on the bed to prevent any soiling
- Inform patient where the commode is and the nurse should be close with the patient if he/she needs to use a bedpan
- Ensure there is adequate lighting and sufficient exposure of the buttocks to prevent any accidental injury.

During the procedure

- Put gloves and apron on
- Lubricate 5 cm of the nozzle of the enema with the water-soluble lubricant (Rushing, 2003)

⌘ Expel all air from the container
⌘ Gently insert the nozzle into the anus to a distance of about 7.5–10 cm into the rectum
⌘ Slowly administer the fluid by rolling the bag from the bottom end while ensuring that there is no backflow
⌘ When the medication has been administered, remove the nozzle and wipe the anus
⌘ Reposition the patient into a comfortable position.

Post-procedure

⌘ Dispose of equipment
⌘ Assist patient with hygiene as necessary
⌘ Document the administration of the enema
⌘ Monitor and report bowel action.

Administration for suppositories

Equipment required

⌘ Disposable apron and gloves
⌘ Disposable wipes/toilet tissues, soap and water/towels
⌘ Disposable incontinence sheets to protect the bed
⌘ Suppositories as prescribed
⌘ Water-soluble lubricant
⌘ Toileting facilities, such as commode or bedpan.

Specific patient preparation required

⌘ Follow above steps as for the administration of an enema.

During the procedure

⌘ Put apron and gloves on
⌘ Open the package
⌘ Lubricate the suppository with a water-soluble lubricant
⌘ Separate buttocks to expose the anus
⌘ Insert the suppository pointed end first and push until it passes the anal sphincter of the rectum (approximately 2–3 cm in adults). If the suppository has not passed this point, it will come out
⌘ Wipe away any excess lubricant.

Post-procedure

⌘ Dispose of any equipment
⌘ Instruct patient to remain lying down for about 15 minutes to avoid rejecting the suppository
⌘ Document the administration of the medication
⌘ Assist patient with toileting and hygiene needs
⌘ Monitor and report bowel action as necessary.

Administration of medications via the vaginal route

Medications for administration via the vaginal route are available in many forms as pessaries and creams.

Pre-procedure

Equipment required

⌘ Disposable tray
⌘ Prescribed medications and applicator if recommended
⌘ Disposable gloves
⌘ Water-soluble lubricant
⌘ Sanitary pad
⌘ Disposal bag
⌘ Adequate lighting.

Specific patient preparation required

⌘ Position patient in either the recumbent or the left lateral position
⌘ In the recumbent position, the patient lies on her back with her knees drawn up and separated and the sides of her feet resting on the bed
⌘ In the left lateral position, the patient lies on her left side with her knees flexed and her buttocks near the edge of the bed
⌘ The patient is encouraged to empty her bladder
⌘ Advise the patient that some of the drug may liquefy and drain out.

During the procedure

⌘ Put on disposable gloves
⌘ Remove medication from wrapper (if applicable)

- Apply lubrication as necessary
- Part the labia majora and insert the medication into the vagina
- A pessary is usually inserted along the posterior vaginal wall and into the top of the vagina
- If using an applicator, insert the barrel of the applicator into the vagina and squeeze the tube to insert the drug while holding the applicator steady. Withdraw the applicator after all the drug has been inserted
- Place the sanitary pad over the vulval area.

Post-procedure

- Document the administration of the medication
- Advise patient to stay lying down for 20 minutes after insertion of the medication
- Dispose of equipment following local policy.

Student skill laboratory activity

- Check a prescription chart for a drug that is to be administered following local policy
- Identify the equipment you would require to administer medication via the different routes
- Prepare the equipment for the specific route in which the drugs are going to be administered
- Identify sites for different types of injection on a manikin
- Practise administering medication via the different routes.

References

Belanger MC (1985) Long-acting neuroleptics: technique for intramuscular injection. *Can Nurse* **81**(8): 41–4

Beyea S, Nicoll L (1996) Back to basics. Administering IM injections the right way. *Am J Nurs* **96**(1): 34–5

Bolander VR (1994) *Sorensen and Luckmann's Basic Nursing. A Psychophysiological Approach*. 3rd edn. WB Saunders, Philadelphia

Burden M (2003) Diabetes: treatment and complications: the nurse's role. *Nurs Times* **99**(2): 30

Craven RF, Hirnle CJ (1996) *Fundamentals of Nursing. Human Health and Function*. 2nd edn. Lippincott, New York

Greenway K (2004) Using the ventrogluteal site for intramuscular injection. *Nurs Stand* **18**(25): 39–42

James A (2004) The legal and clinical implications of crushing tablet medication. *Nurs Times* **11**(50): 28–9

John A, Stevenson T (1995) A basic guide to the principles of drug therapy. *Br J Nurs* **4:** 1194–8

McConnell EA (2000) Administering an intradermal injection. *Nursing* **30**(3): 17

McConnell EA (2001) Clinical do's and don't's: applying nitroglycerin ointment. *Nursing* **31**(6): 17

Nursing and Midwifery Council (2004) *Guidelines for the Administration of Medicines*. NMC, London

Parboteeah S (2002) Safety in practice. In: Hogston R, Simpson P, eds. *Foundations of Nursing Practice. Making the Difference*. Palgrave Macmillan, Bath

Porter-Jones G (2000) Nebulizers – 1: Preparation. *Nurs Times* **96**(36): 45–6

Pulling R (1992) The right place. *Can Nurse* **88**(2): 29–30

Rettig FM, Southby JR (1982) Using different body positions to reduce discomfort from dorsogluteal injection. *Nurs Res* **31**: 219–21

Royal College of Nursing (2000) *Good Practice in Infection Control. Guidance for Nursing Staff*. RCN, London

Royal College of Nursing (2004) *Starting Insulin Treatment in Adults with Type 2 Diabetes: RCN Guidance for Nurses*. RCN, London

Rushing J (2003) Clinical do's and don't's: administering an enema to an adult. *Nursing* **33**(11): 28

Shepherd M (2002) Professional development. Medicines: 3. Managing medicines. *Nurs Times* **98**(17): 43–6

Taylor SJ (1989) A guide to enteral feeding. *Prof Nurse* **4**: 195–200

Walker S (2003) Management of allergic rhinitis. *Nurs Times* **99**(23): 60

Wood L, Wilbourne J, Kyne-Grzebalski D *et al* (2002) Administration of insulin by injection. *Pract Diabetes Int* **19**(Suppl 2): S1–4

Workman B (1999) Safe injection techniques. *Nurs Stand* **13**(39): 47–53

Zenk K (1993) Air bubble. Beware of overdose. *Nursing* **23**: 28–9

Further reading

Addison R (2000) How to administer enemas and suppositories. *Nurs Times* **96**(Suppl 6): 3–4

Henry C (1999) The advantages of using suppositories. *Nurs Times* **95**(17): 50–1

Hill J (2003) Devices for insulin administration. *Nurs Times* **99**(15): 51–2

MacGabhann L (1996) A comparison of two depot injection techniques. *Nurs Stand* **12**(37): 39–41

McGowan S, Wood A (1990) Administering heparin subcutaneously: an evaluation of techniques used and bruising at the site. *Aust J Adv Nurs* **7**(2): 31–9

Moppett S (2000) Which way is up for a suppository? *NT Plus* **96**(19): 12–13

Moppett S, Parker M (1999) Insertion of a suppository. *Nurs Times* **95**(23): suppl 1–2

Rodger MA, King L (2000) Drawing up and administering intramuscular injections: a review of the literature. *J Adv Nurs* **31**: 574–82

Taylor C, Lillis C, Le Mone P (1993) *Fundamentals of Nursing: The Art and Science of Nursing Care*. 2nd edn. JB Lippincott, Philadelphia PA

Thomas A, Shepherd E (1999) To the point. Practical procedures article on the insertion of suppositories. *Nurs Times* **95**(27): 18

Winslow EH (1997) Just how illegible are physicians' medical orders? *Am J Nurs* **97**(9): 66

Chapter 4

Respiratory system

Administration of Entonox

Entonox is an analgesic that is widely used in clinical practice where pain is predictable and of short duration. It provides pain relief for short procedures, such as when changing wound dressings, or during uncomfortable procedures. Entonox is a gaseous mixture of 50% oxygen and 50% nitrous oxide, which is administered via inhalation. Maze and Fujinaga (2000) suggest that inhaled Entonox triggers the release of noradrenergic substances, which activates receptors within the pain pathway preventing signals from reaching the brain. The action of Entonox may start after a few breaths or within 2 minutes of inhalation (British Oxygen Company (BOC), 2001).

Reasons for the procedure

Entonox is recommended for use for the following reasons:

⌘ It reduces the requirement for strong analgesics (opiates) for short procedures
⌘ It reduces side-effects such as nausea and vomiting associated with opiate use
⌘ It has a rapid onset and a short duration.

Pre-procedure

Equipment required

⌘ Entonox is available in cylinders and should be stored at $\geq 6°C$. If the Entonox is stored in temperatures $< 6°C$, the nitrous oxide will separate from the mixture and become less effective
⌘ The gas is delivered using a demand valve, which is activated by the inspiratory effort of the user
⌘ Check the amount of gas in the cylinder before commencing therapy in order to prevent running out of gas during the procedure
⌘ Check that the cylinder is turned on fully
⌘ Use the demand valve test button to ensure that the gas is flowing
⌘ Place an appropriate filter between the patient and the system to prevent infection
⌘ Entonox cylinders should not be lubricated with grease or oil (BOC, 1995)
⌘ Follow health and safety guidelines and local protocols.

Specific patient preparation required

⌘ Identify contraindications (*Box 4.1*)

Box 4.1: Contraindications to the use of Entonox

Artificial, traumatic or spontaneous pneumothorax

Gross abdominal distension

Air embolism

Decompression sickness

Head injury and subsequent impaired consciousness

Alcohol or drug intoxication

Maxillofacial injuries

From Street (2000)

⌘ It is vital that the patient cooperates with this procedure
⌘ The nurse should therefore explain to the patient what the gas does and instruct what he/she has to do
⌘ Give the patient an opportunity to practise a few breaths to ensure that he/she can manage the equipment and technique before commencing the procedure. Self-administration depends on adequate inspiration by the patient
⌘ Ensure that the patient is comfortable and relaxed
⌘ Select mask/mouthpiece depending on the patient's preference. The patient should be advised to hold the mask firmly over the nose and mouth. If using a mouthpiece, the patient should be instructed to hold the mouthpiece between the teeth and sealing around it using the lips
⌘ Familiarize the patient with the noise made on inspiration
⌘ Advise patient/relatives not to smoke.

During the procedure

⌘ Ensure equipment is functioning properly
⌘ Instruct patient to hold the mask/mouthpiece and to breathe normally
⌘ Allow patient to breathe the gas for about 2 minutes before commencing the procedure
⌘ Do not hold the mask on the patient's face
⌘ Assess the patient during the procedure observing for side-effects (*Box 4.2*)
⌘ At all times, the patient should be able to obey commands.

Box 4.2: Side-effects of using short-term Entonox

Light-headedness

Dry mouth

Nausea

Tingling in the fingers

From Street (2000)

Post-procedure

* Assess the patient's pain using agreed protocols
* Record the length of time the gas was administered
* Observe the patient until fully alert
* A short period of rest should be encouraged while the sedative effect wears off
* BOC (1992) recommends that patients should not operate machinery or drive for at least 12 hours
* Follow local decontamination procedures to disinfect the equipment.

Continuous positive airway pressure

Continuous positive airway pressure (CPAP) is a form of respiratory support for the spontaneously breathing patient who is hypoxic (low PaO_2) and may also be hypercapnic (high PCO_2) (Douglas and Engleman, 1999). CPAP may be delivered by continuous flow or by demand flow.

Continuous flow

Gas flows through the system continuously throughout the respiratory cycle. These systems are extremely noisy. They use large volumes of piped gases.

Demand flow

Gas is only allowed to flow when inspiration is initiated by the patient, and is stored in a reservoir from which the patient draws his breath. The patient has to open the valve in order to receive the gas flow. This may increase the patient's respiratory work and so he/she may tire more easily. The amount of continuous positive pressure that the patient receives is determined by the valve attached to the mask. Patients can receive low (2.5–7.5 cm H_2O) or high (10–20 cm H_2O) values of positive end expiratory pressure (PEEP).

Establishing CPAP requires time, patience, effort, motivation, knowledge, understanding and a partnership of trust and safety between nurse and patient.

Both methods require the patient to wear a tight-fitting mask that may be extremely uncomfortable and frightening. CPAP can be delivered through a nasal mask as opposed to a full face mask, but mouth breathing can result in a significant loss of positive pressure in the airways.

Reasons for the procedure

- Acute hypoxaemia without carbon dioxide retention, that is those patients having problems with oxygenation and not with ventilation
- Basal lung collapse
- Fluid overload causing pulmonary oedema
- Patients with COPD may also benefit from CPAP but have to be carefully selected
- Weaning from mechanical ventilation (Woodrow, 2003).

Pre-procedure

Equipment required

- Flow generator
- Oxygen analyzer
- Warm water humidifier
- Elephant tubing
- PEEP valves of 20 cm H_2O
- PEEP valves of 5 cm H_2O
- Face mask and head strap.

Specific patient preparation required

- Position the patient sitting as upright as possible
- Reassure the patient that staff will be observing them closely
- Place the mask on the patient's face before starting CPAP so he/she can anticipate how tight the mask will be applied
- In some areas it may be policy to pass a nasogastric tube to prevent aspiration.

During the procedure

⌘ Inform and explain to the patient and family the rationale for the initiation of CPAP therapy. Check patient's baseline observations, including blood gas analysis
⌘ Turn the flow generator on:
    – increase the flow rate to hear an audible gas flow
    – adjust oxygen concentration to the prescribed levels
    – ensure the correct prescription of PEEP valve is *in situ*
⌘ Turn the warm water humidifier on (refer to the humidification system), ensuring the humidifier contains water to the appropriate level
⌘ Place the mask over the patient's face, explaining the procedure as it happens to the patient – two people may be beneficial
⌘ Apply head strap to mask, aim for a tight seal, without excessive discomfort to the patient or the detriment of their skin integrity.

Post-procedure

⌘ Check seal to ensure no leaks via the mask
⌘ Observe for skin changes as a result of pressure
⌘ Observe for potential complications of CPAP (*Box 4.3*).

Box 4.3: Potential complications of CPAP	
Gastric distention and vomiting	Caused by patient swallowing large amounts of air
Hypotension	Increased intrathoracic pressure and decreased venous return
Patient intolerance	May feel unpleasant and more difficult to breathe. Can feel claustrophobic
Aspiration	Patient may vomit and be unable to remove mask

Oxygen therapy

Oxygen is essential for life — all body tissues need oxygen to survive. Atmospheric air contains approximately 21% oxygen. In a healthy individual, breathing the air supplies the body with adequate oxygen; however, patients may be compromised and require supplementary oxygen in the form of oxygen therapy.

Reasons for the procedure

Oxygen is given to correct hypoxaemia (deficiency of oxygen in arterial blood) and to prevent hypoxia (a lack of oxygen in the tissues). Hypoxia will result in cell death within 3 minutes (Bateman and Leach, 1998).

Pre-procedure

Equipment required

⌘ A prescription for oxygen stating the percentage to be given for what length of time and when the prescription should be reviewed
⌘ An oxygen source: gas cylinder, piped oxygen (in hospital), oxygen concentrator
⌘ Flow meter with control
⌘ Select the appropriate mask/oxygen-delivery device (*Box 4.4*)

Box 4.4: Oxygen delivery devices

Nasal cannulae	Usually used for a low flow rate
Venturi oxygen masks	Used for accurately delivering low concentrations of oxygen of 24%, 28%, 35%, 40% and 60%
Simple oxygen mask	Used to deliver an increased oxygen percentage
Non-rebreathe masks	Allow high concentrations of oxygen to be delivered up to 95% at flow rates of 12 litres/minute

From American Heart Association (1997)

⌘ Oxygen tubing
⌘ Humidification if required.

Specific patient preparation required

⌘ Sit the patient as upright as possible to maximize lung expansion unless contraindicated, such as in hypovolaemic shock and unconsciousness
⌘ Explain and reinforce the significance of keeping the oxygen delivery device *in situ*.

During the procedure

⌘ Assemble equipment for the delivery of the accurate concentration of oxygen. Follow manufacturer's guidelines for accurate setting of oxygen concentration as these may differ

⌘ Assist the patient to secure the mask/cannulae

⌘ Switch on the flow meter to the prescribed concentration.

Post-procedure

⌘ Periodic check of oxygen saturations with a pulse oximeter (see 'Pulse oximetry', Chapter 2)

⌘ Titrate oxygen percentage according to the results of investigation

⌘ Document date and time that oxygen has been commenced

⌘ Monitor patient as necessary (respiratory rate, depth and rhythm, oximetry, arterial blood gases as required)

⌘ Offer mouth and nasal care to prevent drying of mucosa

⌘ Monitor for pressure ulcers caused by the oxygen tubing and mask (bridge of the nose, ear lobe and face)

⌘ Advise patients and relatives regarding the hazards of oxygen therapy

⌘ Monitor for complications of oxygen therapy in chronic respiratory disorders, such as chronic obstructive pulmonary disease, and report to medical staff

⌘ Discuss with the patient potential limitations to activities of living

⌘ Change oxygen mask/cannulae as necessary to prevent infection and as local policy and protocol dictate.

Student skill laboratory activity

⌘ Assemble the equipment to administer via a nasal cannula, Venturi mask, simple oxygen mask and non-rebreathe mask

⌘ Practise putting the devices on a colleague, and discuss your experiences.

Peak flow recording

A peak flow recording measures the maximum flow rate of a forced expiration. It is an effort-dependent test that is generally used as an assessment tool for patients with a respiratory condition. The subsequent results of a peak flow recording are of great relevance in the management of a patient's condition. To identify the variability of the airway obstruction, measurements can be serially recorded (Booker, 2003a).

Reasons for the procedure

✺ An objective assessment of the severity of bronchoconstriction (Baird, 2001)
✺ To monitor asthma on an ongoing basis as part of an action plan by comparing and contrasting the 'best ever' peak flowing recording with the most recent
✺ To monitor the effectiveness of treatment regimens.

Pre-procedure

Equipment required

✺ Peak flow meter (usually Mini-Wright) (preferably the patient's own, if available)
✺ Disposable mouthpiece
✺ Recording chart.

Specific patient preparation required

✺ Position the patient to sitting or standing upright to allow for good chest expansion (Jevon et al, 2000; Nicol et al, 2000; Booker, 2003a) (It may be useful to demonstrate the correct technique initially)
✺ Ensure that the patient is physically able to perform the peak expiratory flow. The patient should be rested or not have undertaken physical exertion (Nicol et al, 2000)
✺ Establish whether the patient is physically able to produce a measurement (*Box 4.5*).

Box 4.5: Reasons for difficulty with performing peak flow

The patient is acutely/severely breathless

Poor coordination	The patient is physically unable to sequence events or hold the peak flow metre steadily
Facial palsy and loose-fitting teeth	Difficult in attaining an adequate seal
Unable to position self appropriately	

During the procedure

✺ Follow manufacturer's instructions for the use of the peak flow meter
✺ Ensure that the cursor is placed back to zero so that a false reading is not obtained

⌘ Check the position of the patient, advise the patient if he/she is physically able to straighten his/her head and neck, and to look straight ahead to maximize air flow (Booker, 2003a)

⌘ Ask the patient to hold the peak flow meter horizontally and advise the patient to take a deep breath in; the patient should then attain a good seal around the disposable mouthpiece. Place the patient's lips around and teeth between the disposable mouthpiece

⌘ The patient should then be asked to breathe out as hard and as fast as possible. This is because the peak flow measures the air flow in the first tenth of a second of a forced blow (Fehrenbach, 1998). Any delay between inhalation and exhalation can reduce the peak flow reading and results can be misleading. Note the measurement by recording the number where the pointer stops (litres/minute). Ask the patient to repeat the procedure another two times as their condition allows. There should be less than 30 litres/minute difference between them (Booker, 2003a).

Post–procedure

⌘ Take the best of the three measurements and document on a recording chart (*Figure 4.1*)
⌘ Consider the factors that may influence the result of the measurement (*Box 4.6*)
⌘ Compare the peak flow measurement with the baseline of the patient's 'best ever'
⌘ Note if the patient experienced any distress during the procedure, such as coughing
⌘ Report to medical staff if results are not within the predicted peak flow range for that individual patient or are deteriorating (*Figure 4.2*)
⌘ Administer medication as per instruction.

Box 4.6: Factors that may influence a peak flow measurement

Gender, age, musculature and body build of the patient

Diurnal variation	The peak flow is significantly lower in the morning than in the evening (Booker, 2003b)
Bronchodilators	The patient may have received medication to promote dilation of the bronchioles, and therefore a peak flow recording pre-medication may be different to post-medication
Chronic respiratory conditions	Irreversible airway obstruction
Position of patient	Lower reading if the patient is lying or sitting down

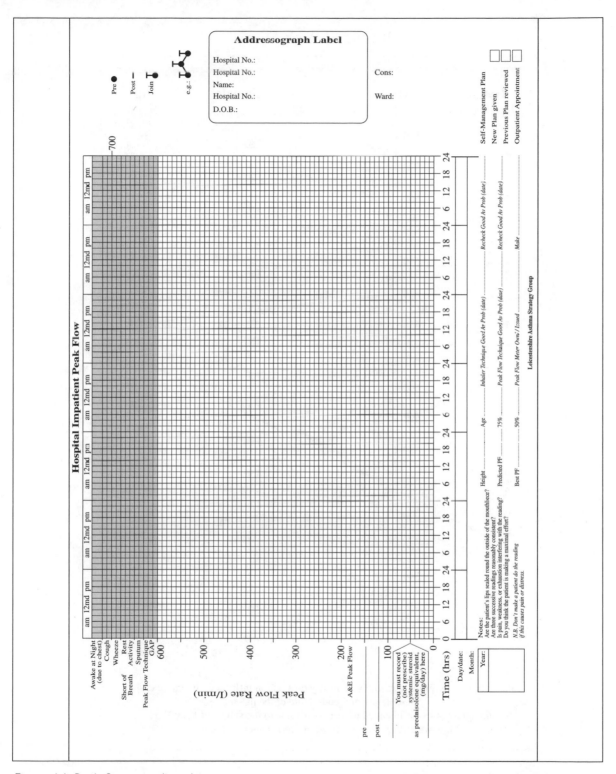

Figure 4.1: Peak flow recording chart

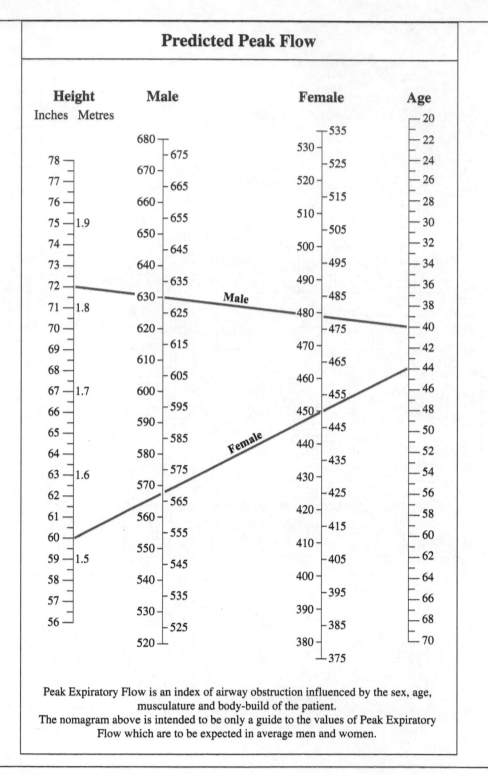

Figure 4.2: Predicted peak flow

Student skill laboratory activity

⌘ Identify the equipment required to undertake a peak flow recording

⌘ Practise measuring and recording your own peak flow while lying, sitting and standing up

⌘ Compare your results with *Figure 4.2*

⌘ How would you instruct another person to undertake a peak flow recording?

Pleural aspiration

In pleural aspiration a needle is introduced through the intercostal space into the pleural cavity between the visceral and parietal pleura in order to remove fluid from the pleural space. A collection of fluid in the pleural space is known as pleural effusion, and this may be caused by a number of diseases such as tuberculosis, malignancy, cardiac failure and kidney failure.

Reasons for the procedure

⌘ For diagnostic purposes – to establish the cause of the effusion
⌘ To relieve breathlessness
⌘ To prevent pleural thickening
⌘ To prevent the development of an empyema after a pneumonic pleural effusion
⌘ To obliterate the pleural space in malignant effusion by injecting substances that produce an inflammatory reaction after aspiration of fluid
⌘ To introduce medication.

Pre-procedure

Equipment required

⌘ Dressing pack
⌘ Pre-labelled specimen pots:
  – cytology
  – microbiology
⌘ Antiseptic skin-cleansing lotion according to local policy
⌘ Local anaesthetic as prescribed

⌘ Syringes and needles for administration of local anaesthetic
⌘ Sterile disposable scalpel
⌘ Protective clothing: goggles, apron and sterile gloves
⌘ Sterile dressing
⌘ Hypoallergenic adhesive tape
⌘ Sterile aspiration pack, which includes:
  – aspiration needle
  – 50 ml Luer-Lok syringe
  – three-way tap
  – connection tubing
  – collection bag
⌘ Specimen request form.

Specific patient preparation of patient

⌘ X-rays of the chest to identify the area to be aspirated
⌘ Assist the patient into a sitting position, resting forward on a bed table for support as this will facilitate the insertion of the aspiration needle between the fifth or sixth intercostal space in the midaxillary line, which is in the posterior and basal part of the chest (Noble et al, 2001). Reinforce the need to let the doctor know of any pain, breathlessness or need to cough during the procedure
⌘ Record the patient's blood pressure, pulse, temperature, respiration rate and oxygen saturation levels as a baseline measurement
⌘ Administer sedation and/or analgesia if required.

During the procedure

⌘ Open the sterile dressing pack on to the trolley
⌘ Add the sterile gloves, syringes and scalpel
⌘ Pour the antiseptic skin-cleansing solution into a receiver. The doctor will put on the goggles, apron and sterile gloves
⌘ Open the remaining equipment onto the trolley
⌘ Expose aspiration site and support patient as necessary
⌘ Assist with the administration of local anaesthetic
⌘ Open the pleural aspiration pack or individual components onto the trolley
⌘ Assist the doctor with the aspiration procedure
⌘ When requested by the doctor, the nurse will hold the specimen bottles under the three-way tap to collect the required specimen(s) so that samples can be sent for cytology and microbiology
⌘ Further free drainage will be collected in the bag
⌘ Once the procedure is complete, the needle will be withdrawn and an appropriate dressing applied.

Post-procedure

⌘ Discard all clinical waste as per local policy
⌘ Record the patient's blood pressure, pulse, temperature, respiration rate and oxygen saturation levels post-procedure
⌘ Document the procedure in the notes
⌘ Ensure the final amount of aspirate is recorded
⌘ Encourage the patient to report any breathlessness or difficulty breathing
⌘ A chest X-ray may be requested to eliminate a pneumothorax (Noble et al, 2001)
⌘ Check the aspiration site daily to ensure that it is not leaking and to ensure healing is taking place
⌘ Send specimens with the request form to the appropriate laboratory.

Sputum sample

A sputum specimen is the collection of a clean, uncontaminated sample of mucus from the respiratory system. Mucus production is necessary to ensure the airways are kept moist and it traps dust and bacteria, enabling the expulsion of foreign bodies. Pathological changes result in an increased production of mucus, which may contain blood, microorganisms and abnormal cells (Maestrelli et al, 2001; Jeffrey and Zhu, 2002). A sputum sample may be collected at a specific time in order to accurately identify certain species of microorganisms.

Reasons for the procedure

⌘ To determine a particular disease process or infection.

Pre-procedure

Equipment required

⌘ Pre-labelled sterile sample container
⌘ Apron
⌘ Gloves
⌘ Mask (if necessary)
⌘ Specimen request form
⌘ Mouthwash
⌘ Tissues.

Specific patient preparation required

❋ Ask patient to clean teeth or remove dentures or provide mouth care (brushing teeth or removing dentures along with rinsing the mouth are attempts to decrease nasopharyngeal flora (Flournoy and Galarza, 2002))
❋ Offer analgesics (Bonde et al, 2002)
❋ Explain to the patient how to expectorate and collect the specimen, differentiating between saliva and mucus
❋ Ensure that the patient is sitting as upright as possible.

During the procedure

❋ Put on gloves, apron and mask (if appropriate)
❋ Encourage patient to take a few deep breaths in before obtaining the specimen as this can loosen mucus secretions (Semple and Elley, 1998)
❋ Once there is a momentum of repeated breaths ask the patient to make a forceful cough and bring up the sputum in his/her mouth
❋ Holding the sterile container to the patient's lips, encourage expectoration of mucus into the container (if able, allow the patient to hold sputum pot)
❋ Observe and note type and consistency of sputum (*Box 4.7*)

Box 4.7: Considerations of sputum consistency and colour

Consistency	Colour and indicative pathology
Mucoid	Greenish yellow — infection
Purulent	Clear/frothy/blood stained — heart failure
Mucopurulent	Reddish brown — lung cancer
Frothy	
Viscous	
Blood stained	

From Law (2000)

❋ Replace lid
❋ Offer mouth care.

Post-procedure

⌘ Remove gloves, apron and mask, and dispose according to local policy
⌘ Put date and time on specimen container and request form
⌘ Place container and request form in the appropriate microbiology bag and transfer to laboratory according to local policy
⌘ Document collection of the specimen in the patient notes.

Suctioning

Suctioning is the drawing of air out of a space to create a vacuum that will then suck in surrounding liquids (Griggs, 1998). Suctioning can be a potentially harmful procedure, resulting in complications including tracheal trauma, suctioning-induced hypoxaemia, hypertension, cardiac arrhythmias and raised intracranial pressure (Joanna Briggs Institute, 2000).

Suctioning should not be performed without a comprehensive respiratory and cardiovascular assessment of the patient, including rate, depth, pattern of breathing as well as pulse oximetry, heart rate and blood pressure.

Reasons for the procedure

⌘ To remove pulmonary secretions
⌘ Maintain a patent airway
⌘ Reduce distress
⌘ Remove small foreign objects.

Pre-procedure

Equipment required

⌘ Individually packed sterile disposable gloves
⌘ Clean disposable glove
⌘ Bottle of sterile water (label when open and dispose of after 24 hours)
⌘ Sterile water
⌘ Suction unit
⌘ Suction catheters – calculate size of catheter by dividing tube size by 2 and multiplying the result by 3 (Griggs, 1998)

⌘ Sputum trap (if required)
⌘ Clinical waste bag
⌘ Sterile disposable dish.

Specific patient preparation required

⌘ Consider whether pre-oxygenation is required
⌘ Emphasize the need for patient cooperation.

During the procedure

⌘ Check the suction pressure on the wall-mounted suction device
⌘ Recommended pressure: 14–16 kPa (kilopascal); 100–120 mmHg low pressure (Regan, 1988; Martin, 1989)
⌘ Switch the suction unit on
⌘ Check suction working (by placing thumb over end of tubing you should feel suction, and the dial on the flow meter should bounce upwards)
⌘ Pour sterile water into disposable dish
⌘ Attach the end of the suction catheter to the suction tubing. Keep the rest of the catheter in the sterile pack, either hold in non-dominant hand or place under arm and hold close to chest
⌘ Place a clean disposable glove on the hand that will be controlling the catheter (usually the dominant hand)
⌘ Keeping the suction catheter sterile, withdraw from packaging
⌘ Introduce catheter into tracheostomy, advance approximately two-thirds of the catheter, no further than the carina (resistance will be felt) to minimize trauma
⌘ Pull back catheter a small way (1–3 cm) and apply suction by placing a finger on the hole or Y connection
⌘ Withdraw all of the catheter on constant suction
⌘ The procedure should take no longer than 10 seconds (Fiorentini, 1992) to avoid complications (*Box 4.8*)
⌘ Observe sputum type, colour and consistency
⌘ Wrap suction catheter around gloved hand and pull glove over used catheter and discard
⌘ Remove any secretions trapped in suction tubing, place the tip of the tubing into the sterile water until tubing is clear and contained in the suction bottle
⌘ Repeat procedure with a new suction catheter every time until removal of secretions have been achieved, without detriment to patient's condition.

> **Box 4.8: Complications of suctioning**
>
> Tracheal mucosal damage
>
> Hypoxia
>
> Infection
>
> Atelectasis
>
> Paroxysmal coughing
>
> Vagal nerve stimulation

Post-procedure

⌘ Allow the patient a period of recovery time and reassess the need for suctioning, response to suction and the need to repeat the procedure

⌘ For fenestrated trachesotomy tubes, replace fenestrated inner tube with a non-fenestrated inner tube

⌘ Record actions on appropriate documentation.

Use of sputum trap

⌘ You may be instructed to collect a sputum specimen for microbiology purposes

⌘ In order to collect this type of specimen from a tracheostomy, a sputum trap is incorporated within the suction circuit

⌘ Attach the tip of the suction tubing to the rigid prong of the trap

⌘ Attach the suction port of the catheter to the flexible end of the trap

⌘ Use the same technique as described above

⌘ Any sputum will be collected in the container

⌘ Unscrew the lid and replace with the plain lid from the packaging

⌘ Label as per hospital policy and send to laboratory.

Suctioning via a nasopharyngeal airway

⌘ A nasopharyngeal airway may be placed and used for patients with a lot of secretions at the back of the throat but who cannot cough or expectorate (Bennett, 2003).

Equipment required

⌘ As for suctioning a tracheosotomy.

During the procedure

⌘ Mark on the catheter, with gloved finger and thumb, the distance from the patient's earlobe to tip of nose. This ensures the catheter length inserted remains in the pharyngeal area and does not enter the trachea (Bennett, 2003)

⌘ Moisten the suction catheter tip with sterile water to ease the movement of the catheter down the airway

⌘ Proceed as for tracheostomy suctioning.

Post-procedure

❋ As for suctioning a tracheostomy.

Student skill laboratory activity

❋ Familiarize yourself with the various types of suction catheters available to you

❋ Practise suctioning on a manikin.

Tracheostomy care

A tracheostomy is an artificial opening (stoma) in the anterior wall of the trachea, created by making an incision in the neck (Woodrow, 2002). This will allow air to enter the trachea and lungs and bypass the upper airway, which normally filters, warms and humidifies inspired air. A tracheostomy can be temporary or permanent and may be performed as an emergency procedure or as a routine operation.

Reasons for the procedure

A tracheostomy may be performed for the following reasons:

❋ An obstructed airway, such as laryngeal oedema, foreign body
❋ To remove bronchial secretions
❋ In patients having prolonged mechanical ventilation
❋ Shortens the length of stay in an intensive care unit
❋ To prevent aspiration.

Pre-procedure

Equipment required

For cleaning the stoma site:

❋ Gloves
❋ Apron
❋ Dressing trolley

⌘ Dressing pack
⌘ Sterile normal saline
⌘ Dressings with pre-cut hole
⌘ Trachcostomy tapes
⌘ Sterile receive
⌘ Spare tracheostomy tube
⌘ Sterile scissors.

Additional equipment required when changing a tracheostomy tube:

⌘ Tracheal dilators
⌘ Tracheostomy tubes — same size and one smaller size
⌘ Suction unit
⌘ Suction catheters
⌘ Bottle of sterile water
⌘ Sterile bowl
⌘ Waste bag
⌘ Water-based lubrication.

Specific preparation of the patient required for tracheostomy care and change of tracheostomy tube

⌘ The patient needs to lie flat, ideally with his/her neck extended.

During the procedure

1. Tracheostomy care is a two-nurse procedure, which must be carried out aseptically
2. Ensure that the patient continues to receive any ongoing interventions such as oxygen therapy and mechanical assistance with his/her breathing
3. Prepare the trolley and place the equipment required on it
4. Prepare the sterile field to work from
5. If an inner tube is present, this is unlocked and removed. It is then placed into a sterile bowl and rinsed with normal saline
6. A temporary replacement tube is inserted and locked
7. One practitioner securely holds the tube in place and the other practitioner removes the tapes and dressing
8. Assess stoma site and clean by gently swabbing with non-fibre shedding gauze using warmed normal saline
9. The flange of the tube is cleaned to remove any secretions
10. A suitable dressing is placed around the stoma
11. The tracheostomy tube is secured by attaching the flanges of the tube using tracheostomy tapes cut to size (as necessary). The tapes should be tight enough to prevent accidental dislodgement of the tube. The tension can be assessed by ensuring that two fingers can slide between the tapes and the neck (Serra, 2000).

Changing a tracheostomy tube

⌘ Usually the first change of a tracheostomy tube is undertaken by medical staff; this occurs 3–5 days after surgery.

During the procedure

1. Follow previous procedure stages 1–4
2. Test the integrity of the cuff by inflating and deflating it
3. Suction the tracheostomy (see 'Suctioning', Chapter 4)
4. Suction the oropharynx
5. Place suction catheter past the lumen of the tracheostomy tube and suction while the cuff is deflated
6. Ask the patient to take a deep breath and remove the tube using an anticlockwise turning motion on expiration. If the stoma closes and the patient is unable to breathe, tracheal dilators may be required to keep the stoma open until a tracheostomy tube has been inserted
7. Inspect the stoma for complications (infection, inflammation, tissue necrosis, narrowing, haematoma)
8. Lubricate the tracheostomy tube before insertion
9. Replace with new tracheostomy tube and inflate cuff to produce a seal
10. Check that the airway is patent
11. Place dressings around stoma and secure tracheostomy tube.

Removing a tracheostomy tube

⌘ Follow stages 1–6 as above for 'Changing a tracheostomy tube'
⌘ The stoma should be cleaned, dried and covered with a non-absorbent, water-repellent dressing until the stoma has closed
⌘ The wound should be dressed as required.

Post-procedure

⌘ Monitor respiratory function
⌘ Ensure emergency equipment is available
⌘ Provide communication aids as necessary
⌘ Provide facilities for mouth care
⌘ Document all interventions.

Student skill laboratory activity

⌘ Identify different types of tracheostomy tubes for short-term and long-term use, during mechanical ventilation and for speaking

⌘ Practise inserting and removing the tracheostomy tubes in a manikin.

Underwater water seal drainage

A chest drain is the insertion of a chest tube into the pleural cavity. Inserting a chest drain restores negative pressure that is required for full expansion of the lung and normal respiration.

Reasons for procedure

⌘ To remove accumulated air, blood or fluids from the chest cavity without allowing air to re-enter
⌘ To allow re-expansion of the collapsed lung
⌘ To prevent collapse and compression of the lung (Allibone, 2003).

Pre-procedure

Equipment required

⌘ Dressing trolley
⌘ Minor operations pack/chest insertion packs
⌘ Selection of chest tubes
⌘ Guide wire with dilators for insertion of small tubes
⌘ Skin antiseptic solution
⌘ Sterile drapes
⌘ Sterile gloves and gowns
⌘ Gauze swabs
⌘ A selection of syringes and needles
⌘ Local anaesthetic — 10 ml 2% lidocaine (Tomlinson and Treasure, 1997)
⌘ Scalpel and blade
⌘ Suture '1' silk
⌘ Forceps for blunt dissection
⌘ Sterile connecting tubes
⌘ Closed drainage system (one-bottle system, *Figure 4.3*; two-bottle system, *Figure 4.4;* or plastic multi-chamber units, *Figure 4.5*)

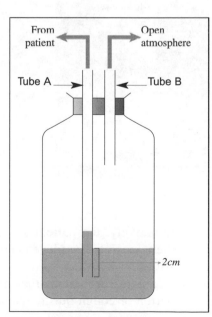

Figure 4.3: One-bottle system

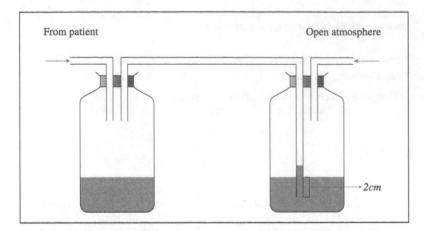

Figure 4.4: Two-bottle underwater chest drain system

From patient

Open atmosphere

2cm

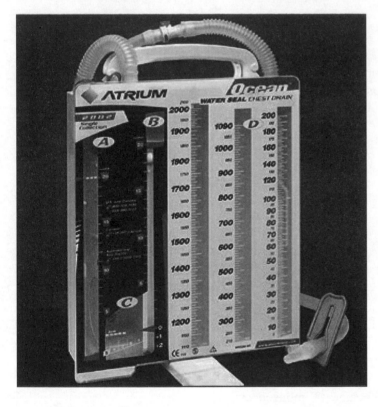

Figure 4.5: Plastic multi-chamber units (reproduced with permission from Atrium Medical Corporation, Hudson, USA)

✱ Two large tube clamps
✱ Sterile water (500 ml)
✱ Clear waterproof dressings.

Specific patient preparation required

✱ Chest X-ray
✱ Baseline observations should be recorded in order to monitor for improvement or deterioration in the condition of the patient
✱ Position of patient — an upright position is required: the patient can be sitting on the edge of the bed with his/her arms crossed and raised to the level of the chin, with arms and head resting on a pillow that is on the bedside table (Avery, 2000); alternatively, the patient should sit upright in the bed with an arm above his/her head. The patient may also be placed in the supine position if his/her condition does not enable an upright position
✱ Explain to the patient that he/she should inform the staff if he/she wishes to move, alter position or cough during the procedure.

During the procedure

- Insertion of the chest tube is carried out by a doctor
- The role of the nurse is to support the patient and to assist the doctor
- Ongoing monitoring of the patient's respiration.

Management of the drainage system using a one-bottle system

- The system must be made safe by ensuring that all connections are airtight and secure
- The connection tube leading from the patient into the bottle (tube A) must be 2–3 cm below the water line in the bottle
- The tube leading from the bottle to the atmosphere (tube B) must be shorter and above the water level
- The bottle should not be raised above the level of the patient's chest, as water can siphon back into the chest cavity
- Observe that the fluid level is fluctuating (if fluctuation is not present, the lung may have expanded or the tube may be blocked (Gallon, 1998))
- Drainage should be monitored and recorded on the fluid balance chart. The frequency will depend on the condition of the patient
- More frequent observations are required in cardiac surgery patients, initially every 30 minutes. If drainage is excessive after cardiac surgery (>100 ml/hr except for the first 3–4 hours post-surgery), inform medical staff (Nelson and Tully, 1998)
- Monitor the colour and consistency of the drainage
- Clamps should only be used when changing bottles and during accidental disconnection
- Regular observations for air leak; listen for sucking noise
- Insertion site should be checked daily for leakage, odour, infection and emphysema
- The tubing should be laid horizontally on the bed before dropping vertically into the drainage bottle (Munnell, 1997; Avery, 2000). The formation of dependent loops will interfere with the drainage, and higher pressure will be required to force air out of the system.

Post-procedure

- The patient should be nursed in the semi-upright position with regular change of position to encourage drainage
- Observations: pulse, blood pressure, arterial blood gases (Avery, 2000), oxygen saturation, respiratory rate, breath sounds, air entry, respiratory pattern, effort and depth
- Mobilization should be encouraged as and when possible
- Huffing and coughing will also force air from the pleural space out through the chest drain (Gallon, 1998)
- Adequate analgesics in the form of opiates (unless contraindicated)
- Observe for complications (*Box 4.9*).

Box 4.9: Complications of chest drain insertion

Tension pneumothorax

Surgical emphysema

Fluid collection in the dependent loop of the tubing (McMahon-Parkes, 1997)

Blocking of tube

Disconnection

Removal of chest drains

✾ Entonox may be used for controlling pain during removal of the chest drain
✾ Patient should be instructed to take three or four breaths and hold his/her breath on deep inspiration
✾ During this time, one nurse quickly pulls the drain out; the assistant ties the purse-string suture and then applies an airtight dressing.

References

Allibone L (2003) Nursing management of chest drains. *Nurs Stand* **17**(22): 45–54

American Heart Association (1997) *Pediatric Advanced Life Support*. AHA, Dallas

Avery S (2000) Insertion and management of chest drains. *NT Plus* **96**(37): 3–6

Baird A (2001) The benefits of recording peak flow. *Practice Nursing* **12**(2): 62–4

Bateman NT, Leach RM (1998) ABC of oxygen. Acute oxygen therapy. *Br Med J* **317:** 798–801

Bennett C (2003) Nursing the breathless patient. *Nurs Stand* **17**(17): 45–51

Bonde P, McManus K, McAnespie M, McGuigan J (2002) Lung surgery: identifying the subgroup at risk for sputum retention. *Eur J Cardiothorac Surg* **22**(1): 18–22

Booker R (2003a) Lung function testing. *Practice Nursing* **14**(4): 175–7

Booker R (2003b) Lung function testing. *Practice Nursing* **14**(3): 127–30

British Oxygen Company (1992) *Data Sheet Revision 2*. BOC Gases, Manchester

British Oxygen Company (1995) *Data Sheet*. BOC Group, Guildford

British Oxygen Company (2001) *Entonox. Controlled Pain Relief. Reference Guide*. BOC Group, Guildford

Douglas N, Engleman H (1999) CPAP therapy: outcomes and patient use. *Thorax* **53**(Suppl 3): S47–8

Fehrenbach C (1998) Chronic obstructive pulmonary disease. *Prof Nurse* **13:** 771–7

Fiorentini A (1992) Potential hazards of tracheo-bronchial suctioning. *Intensive Crit Care Nurs* **8**(4): 217–26

Flournoy D, Galarza L (2002) Does rinsing the mouth before expectoration improve sputum specimen quality? *Chest* **122**(1): 382–3

Gallon A (1998) Pneumothorax. *Nurs Stand* **13**(10): 35–9

Griggs A (1998) Tracheostomy: suctioning and humidification. *Nurs Stand* **13**(2): 49–56

Jeffrey P, Zhu J (2002) Mucin producing elements and inflammatory cells. *Novartis Found Symp* **248:** 51–68

Jevon P, Ewens B, Manzie J (2000) Practical procedures for nurses: measuring peak expiratory flow. *Nurs Times* **96**(38): 49–50

Joanna Briggs Institute (2000) Tracheal suctioning of adults with an artificial airway. *Evidence Based Practice Information Sheets for Health Professionals* **4**(4): 1–6 [available at www.joannabriggs.edu.au/pdf/bpsuc.pdf]

Law C (2000) A guide to assessing sputum. *Nurs Times* **96**(Suppl 24): S7–S10

Maestrelli P, Saetta M, Mapp CE, Fabbri LM (2001) Remodelling response to infection and injury. Airway inflammation and hypersecretion of mucus in smoking subjects with COPD. *Am J Respir Crit Care Med* **164**(10 Pt 2): S76–S80

Martin LK (1989) Management of the altered airway in the head and neck cancer patient. *Semin Oncol Nurs* **5**(3): 182–90

Maze M, Fujinaga M (2000) Recent advances in understanding the actions and toxicity of nitrous oxide. *Anaesthesia* **5**(4): 311–14

McMahon-Parkes K (1997) Management of pleural drains. *Nurs Times* **93**(52): 48–52

Munnell ER (1997) Thoracic drainage. *Ann Thorac Surg* **63:** 1497–502

Nelson S, Tully C (1998) Thoracic surgery. In: Shuldham C, ed. *Cardiorespiratory Nursing*. Stanley Thornes, Cheltenham

Nicol M, Bavin C, Bedford-Turner S, Cronin P, Rawlings-Anderson K (2000) *Essential Nursing Skills*. Mosby, Edinburgh

Noble S, Leach W, Hargreaves P (2001) Improving aspiration technique. *Eur J Palliat Care* **8**(2): 73

Regan H (1988) Tracheal mucosal injury: the nurse's role. *Nursing* **3**(29): 1064–6

Semple M, Elley K (1998) Collecting a sputum specimen. *Nurs Times* **94**(48): suppl 1–2

Serra A (2000) Tracheostomy care. *Nurs Stand* **14**(42): 45–52

Street D (2000) A practical guide to giving Entonox. *Nurs Times* **96**(34): 47–8

Tomlinson MA, Treasure T (1997) Insertion of a chest drain: how to do it. *Br J Hosp Med* **58**(6): 248–52

Woodrow P (2002) Managing patients with a tracheostomy in acute care. *Nurs Stand* **16**(44): 39–46

Woodrow P (2003) Using non-invasive ventilation in acute wards: part 1. *Nurs Stand* **18**(1): 39–44

Further reading

British Medical Association/Royal Pharmaceutical Society Great Britain (2003) *British National Formulary*. BMA/RPSGB, London

Department of Health and Social Security (1985) *Guidelines for Prescribing Long-term Oxygen. National Health Service England and Wales: Amendments to Drug Tariff. DTA/1Z*. DHSS, London

Esmond G, Mikelsons C (2001) Oxygen therapy. In: Esmond G, ed. *Respiratory Nursing*. Bailliere Tindall, London

Godden J, Hiley C (1998) Managing the patient with a chest drain: a review. *Nurs Stand* 12(32): 35–9

Gray E (2000) Pain management for patients with chest drains. *Nurs Stand* 14(23): 40–4

Harkin H (2001) Tracheostomy patient care. *Nurs Times* 97(25): 37–8

Henderson N (1999) Mechanical ventilation. *Nurs Stand* 13(44): 49–53

Medical Research Council Working Party (1981) Long-term domiciliary oxygen therapy in chronic hypoxia cor pulmonale complicating chronic bronchitis and emphysema. *Lancet* i: 681–6

National Institutes of Health, National Heart, Lung and Blood Institute (2001) *Global Strategy for the Diagnosis, Management, and Prevention of Chronic Obstructive Pulmonary Disease*. NHLBI/WHO Workshop Report. NIH, Bethesda MD [Available online at www.goldcopd.com]

Nocturnal Oxygen Therapy Trial Group (1980) Continuous or nocturnal oxygen therapy in hypoxaemic chronic obstructive lung disease. *Ann Intern Med* 93: 391–8

Nursing and Midwifery Council (2002) *Code of Professional Conduct*. NMC, London

Owen S, Gould D (1997) Underwater seal chest drains: the patient's experience. *J Clin Nurs* 6(3): 215–25

Partington JR (1989) *A Short History of Chemistry*. 3rd edn. Dover Publications, New York

Preston R (2001) Introducing non-invasive positive pressure ventilation. *Nurs Stand* 15(26): 42–5

Pryor JA, Webber BA (1998) *Physiotherapy for Respiratory and Cardiac Problems*. Churchill Livingstone, Edinburgh

Restrick LJ, Paul WA, Braid GM *et al* (1993) Assessment and follow up of patients prescribed long-term oxygen treatment. *Thorax* 48: 7708–13

Richardson M (2003) The physiology of mucus and sputum production in the respiratory system. *Nurs Times* 99(23): 63–4

Sealey L (2002) Nurse administration of Entonox to manage pain in ward settings. *Nurs Times* 98(46): 28–9

Tooley C (2002) The management and care of chest drains. *Nurs Times* 98(26): 48–50

Wong D, Pasero CL (1997) Using anaesthetics to control procedural pain. *Am J Nurs* 97(1): 17

Woodrow P (2003) Using non-invasive ventilation in acute wards: part 2. *Nurs Stand* 18(1): 41–4

Chapter 5

Cardiovascular system

Management of arterial lines and catheters

An intra-arterial catheter is a small plastic tube placed in an artery to which monitoring devices are attached. A variety of arterial sites can be used for cannulation; the most readily accessed are the radial artery and the femoral artery (Mawer *et al*, 1999).

Other sites for peripheral artery catheterization may include the posterior tibial artery, ulnar artery and dorsalis pedis.

Reasons for the procedure

- Monitor blood pressure closely
- Arterial blood sampling
- Therapeutic purposes
- Avoids repeated stabbing.

Pre-procedure

Equipment required

- Minor operations pack
- Arterial line insertion kit
- Pressure-monitoring cable and display module
- Pressure transducer set-up
- Disposable pressure infuser bag
- Antiseptic agent as per local policy
- Infusion solution as per local policy or 0.9% normal saline/5000 units heparin
- Occlusive dressing
- Suture
- Local anaesthetic (lidocaine).

Specific patient preparation required

* Patient should be on bed rest
* Procedure must be explained to the patient, and his/her consent must be obtained
* A modified Allen's test must be performed before insertion of the catheter in the radial artery to evaluate collateral circulation (Perry and Potter, 1994; Mawer et al, 1999)
* Identification of non-dominant arm.

During the procedure

* The insertion of an arterial catheter must be performed by a doctor or a person who has undertaken specific training for this role
* Before inserting the catheter, the monitoring equipment is assembled and tested (giving set, transducer, flush device, display monitor, sampling port, three-way tap, pressure bag and the solution as prescribed)
* The insertion of an arterial catheter is an aseptic procedure (Stansby et al, 2003). The doctor must follow local guidelines to prevent contamination
* The nurse supports the patient's arm/hand and may be involved in assisting the doctor
* Once the catheter is *in situ* the arterial line is connected to the monitoring equipment using a Luer-Lok
* The catheter is sutured to prevent accidental displacement
* The site is covered with a clear occlusive dressing
* The peripheral pulse is assessed to ensure circulation of the hand
* A properly functioning arterial line will have the four features shown in *Box 5.1*.

Box 5.1: Features of a functioning arterial line

Blood can be drawn from the catheter

The system can be zeroed

There should be a mechanism to keep the catheter clear

A dependable waveform

From Loach and Thomson (1987)

Post-procedure

* The catheter tip serves as the zero reference point, and the equipment should be calibrated accordingly
* Explain to the patient the need to manage the arm
* Elevate and support limb in a neutral position

- Check for colour and circulation at site and extremities
- Monitor for pain, numbness, bleeding and infection (Way, 2000; Srejic and Wenker, 2003)
- Ask patient not to use the arm; assist with activities of living as necessary
- Ensure there are no air bubbles in the system
- Dispose of equipment as per local policy
- Ensure that arterial line is clearly marked so that drugs cannot be injected via this route.

Removal of catheter

- Check the patient's international normalized ratio (INR)/prothrombin time
- Prepare equipment: sterile tray with cutters, antiseptic agent, gauze squares, clear occlusive dressing
- Inform patient of the procedure
- Disconnect the monitoring equipment
- Cleanse site with antiseptic or as per local policy
- While holding catheter, remove sutures
- Gently withdraw catheter while applying direct pressure
- Apply pressure for about 5–10 minutes until haemostasis has been achieved
- Dressing should be applied
- The site should be assessed every 15 minutes for 1 hour, and limb activity should be minimized for at least 1 hour after removal of the catheter
- Check catheter for clots and ensure that the entire catheter has come out.

Bone marrow aspiration and biopsy

The bone marrow aspiration and biopsy procedure is one of the most valuable diagnostic procedures necessary in order to evaluate haematological disorders. Although medical staff mainly perform this procedure, there are some hospitals where this procedure is performed by specially trained nurse practitioners.

Bone marrow aspiration is a diagnostic procedure undertaken to assess development of blood cells and the cells within the bone marrow for any abnormalities and to establish a diagnosis. Aspiration is the withdrawal of bone marrow fluid to gain information of developing cells. The sites for bone marrow aspiration are listed in *Box 5.2*.

Box 5.2: Safe and preferred sites for bone marrow aspiration and biopsy

Posterior iliac crest (aspiration and biopsy)

Anterior iliac crest (aspiration and biopsy)

Sternum (aspiration only)

Reasons for the procedure

⌘ Unexplained thrombocytopenia (abnormally low platelet count)
⌘ Pancytopenia (simultaneous decrease in red cells, white cells and platelets)
⌘ Diagnostic purposes
⌘ Monitor effectiveness of treatment
⌘ Abnormal cells in peripheral blood
⌘ Metastatic disease
⌘ Chromosomal abnormality
⌘ Immunodeficiency syndrome
⌘ Fever of unknown origin (Trewhitt, 2001).

Pre-procedure

Equipment required

⌘ Clean trolley
⌘ Dressing pack
⌘ Cleaning solution (chlorhexadine gluconate 0.5% in alcohol 70%)
⌘ 3 x 10 ml syringes
⌘ 23- and 25-gauge needles
⌘ Sterile gloves
⌘ The following pre-labelled with patient's data:
   — specimen request form
   — frosted slide
   — formalin histology pot
   — cytogenic universal container
   — EDTA bottle
⌘ Bone marrow aspirate needle
⌘ Trephine needle
⌘ 10 ml 1% or 2% lidocaine solution (Copp, 2001a; Trewhitt, 2001)
⌘ Sharps box.

The nurse must prepare the trolley using an aseptic technique, which needs to be practised throughout.

Specific patient preparation required

⌘ No clinical preparation is necessary for the procedure unless the patient has abnormal blood counts, such as low platelets or abnormal INR. If the patient is on anticoagulation therapy, it needs to be stopped 2 days before the procedure. The INR needs to be checked on the day and needs to be under 1.5; the medical staff need to review the platelet and INR count in order to prevent bleeding problems during the procedure

⌘ A medication history is obtained from the patient

⌘ Promote relaxation and a calm atmosphere as these will help the patient cope with the procedural pain

⌘ Expose site to aspiration (*Box 5.2*).

During the procedure

⌘ A second person is required to ensure the safe collection of specimens and to support the patient through the procedure

⌘ Assist the patient into a position to enable access for sternal puncture (supine) or anterior or posterior iliac crest puncture (lateral position) (*Box 5.2*)

⌘ Palpate the iliac crest and select a site where it is closest to the skin

⌘ Mark the aspiration site with a pen (*Box 5.2*)

⌘ Open the dressing pack, ensuring that a sterile field is maintained

⌘ Open the necessary equipment onto the sterile field

⌘ Clean the skin using an antiseptic solution

⌘ Put on sterile gloves

⌘ Local anaesthetic is drawn up, injected into the subcutaneous tissue using a 26-gauge needle and into the surface of the bone using a 23-gauge needle (Copp, 2001a); allow 5 minutes for the local anaesthetic to take effect

⌘ The obturator is inserted into the aspirate needle and locked

⌘ The aspirate needle is then inserted by holding the capped end firmly in the palm of the hand until it pierces the cortex of the bone. The bone is hard to puncture and therefore pressure has to be exerted; once the obturator reaches the bone marrow there is reduced resistance

⌘ Unlock the cap and remove the obturator. Quickly attach a 10 ml syringe to the needle so that 0.5–1 ml sample fluid is drawn from the bone marrow (Copp, 2001b)

⌘ The needle is removed and direct pressure is applied until bleeding stops. The site is covered with a sterile dressing.

Preparation of the specimens/slides

⌘ The biopsy is then placed in the relevant container for investigation (Copp, 2001c)

⌘ One drop of aspirate is deposited onto a slide(s). Using a clear slide, the drop of aspirate is spread across the slide. Allow slide(s) to dry.

Post-procedure

⌘ Encourage patient to lie on his/her back for 10–15 minutes to prevent any further bleeding

⌘ Disassemble equipment and dispose of sharps in the sharps bin

⌘ Check bone marrow site for signs of bleeding. If there are no signs, the patient can start mobilizing

- ⌘ Offer analgesia as this procedure can be painful
- ⌘ Send specimens to the appropriate laboratory
- ⌘ Document date and time of procedure.

Blood component transfusion

This procedure involves the administration of red blood cells and plasma components (fresh frozen plasma, cryoprecipitate and platelets). Before commencing the transfusion, a sample of blood is taken for ABO/rhesus D testing and cross-matching. According to the British Committee for Standards in Haematology (2003), 39% of all 'wrong blood' incidents occurred at this stage. Rigorous cross-checking of patient details should be undertaken when obtaining samples for the purposes of cross-matching.

Reasons for the procedure

- ⌘ Severe blood loss (Class 3 and 4 haemorrhage: 1.5–2 litres)
- ⌘ To manage specific deficiency disorders or disease processes.

Pre-procedure

Equipment required

- ⌘ Gloves
- ⌘ Prescription for the transfusion
- ⌘ Blood-giving set
- ⌘ Blood warmer if the adult is receiving more than 50 ml/kg/hour or if the adult has cold agglutinin disease (Royal College of Nursing (RCN), 2004). Follow manufacturer's instructions for use
- ⌘ Electronic infusion pump that has been certified as suitable for blood transfusion. Follow manufacturer's instructions for use
- ⌘ Drip stand
- ⌘ Temperature, pulse, respiration (TPR) and blood pressure (BP) recording chart
- ⌘ Fluid balance chart
- ⌘ Patient's medical notes.

Specific patient preparation required

⌘ Ascertain if the patient has had any previous transfusion or allergies
⌘ Identify cultural beliefs that may influence whether or not the patient receives a transfusion (e.g. Jehovah's Witness)
⌘ An intravenous route should be established using a 20-gauge cannula (Atterbury, 2001)
⌘ Record baseline observations of TPR and BP
⌘ Administer any medication prescribed while the patient is receiving transfusion.

During the procedure

Collection of blood component

⌘ The person asked to collect the blood should check that the details on the blood collection form (issued by the Blood Transfusion Service) match those of the patient's notes and patient's wristband. The following details should be checked: name(s), surname, address, date of birth and hospital number (RCN, 2004)
⌘ Before removing the blood from the fridge, the collector should cross-check the patient's identification details on the blood collection form against the compatibility label on the blood bag to ensure that the correct blood is being collected
⌘ The blood collected should be documented in a register or via an electronic release system, and the date, time and signature of the collector should be noted. Within 30 minutes of the blood being collected from storage, transfusion should be commenced as any longer would facilitate the risk of bacterial growth in the blood (Bradbury and Cruickshank, 2000; RCN, 2004).

Administration of the blood

⌘ Confirm accuracy of blood to be transfused by the patient's bedside; cross-checking the details on the unit of blood with the patient's notes, wristband, blood collection form and prescription chart (Tremayne, 2003)
⌘ Visually check the integrity of the blood to be transfused. Observe for air bubbles and clotting
⌘ Hang the unit of blood to be transfused on the drip stand
⌘ Put on gloves to protect yourself from the blood components
⌘ Using an aseptic technique, part the plastic flaps that protect and cover the entry port to expose it
⌘ Remove the giving set from the pack and turn the flow regulator off (this usually means rolling the wheel in a downward direction)
⌘ Insert the spike inlet of the filtered giving set fully into the container
⌘ Fill the drip chamber with blood by gently squeezing the drip chamber. This will prevent air entry into the tubing during transfusion. The drip chamber should be half full
⌘ The filter chamber above the drip chamber will fill up as a consequence of the above step

✼ Turn the flow regulator on (this usually means rolling the wheel in an upward direction), but not fully — just enough to prime the line
✼ Remove the plastic guard of the connector of the giving set (remembering to maintain asepsis), remove the bung of the cannula (some pressure may have to be put on a vein briefly to stem bleeding) and insert the connector into the bung and screw until firmly in place
✼ Secure the cannula in place with a clear dressing that will enable the nurse to observe for signs of redness, inflammation or extravasation
✼ Set the flow rate of the blood according to prescription.

Post-procedure

✼ Remove gloves and dispose of waste accordingly
✼ Monitor the patient's temperature and pulse 15 minutes after commencement of each unit of the transfusion and record them on the transfusion observation chart
✼ Observe for signs of transfusion reaction (*Box 5.3*)

Box 5.3: Adverse reactions that can occur in a transfusion

Pulmonary oedema	The patient will present with coughing and breathlessness as a consequence of cardiac overload
Acute haemolytic reaction	The patient may present with mild to severe symptoms: chest pain, loin pain, breathlessness, rigors, flushing, oliguria, oozing from wounds or puncture sites, hypotension and tachycardia
Allergic reaction	The patient may present with flushing, itching, rashes, wheezing, chest tightness, urticarial hives and laryngeal oedema as a consequence of plasma proteins in the donor's blood
Infective shock	The patient will present with hypotension and tachycardia as a consequence of bacterial contamination of the blood

---

✼ Ensure that the start and finish of each unit of blood is documented and that a care plan is written and evaluated
✼ While *in situ,* a fluid balance chart should be maintained with the volume of blood entered accordingly
✼ In the event of an adverse reaction, stop the transfusion immediately and inform the doctor or nurse in charge and implement local policy for such a complication
✼ Retain the whole unit in a clinical waste and return to the hospital transfusion laboratory.

Cardiac monitoring

Cardiac monitoring involves the detection and graphical recording of cardiac electrical impulses in order to assess cardiac activity (Marieb, 2004). The continuous monitoring of cardiac rate and rhythm provides the means to anticipate and identify the occurrence of potentially harmful disorders of cardiac rhythm and conduction and to assess the patient's response to any interventions.

There are two basic types of continuous cardiac monitoring. Hard wire monitoring involves the patient being connected via a cable from electrodes placed on his/her chest to a bedside monitor. Telemetry is where the patient carries a battery-powered transducer to relay the signal of the heart rhythm to a receiver that may be some distance away, thus giving the patient more freedom of movement. Abnormal events are sensed by the monitors, and an alarm sounds.

Cardiac monitoring is part of an overall patient assessment and needs to be performed against a background knowledge of the patient's history, treatment (including drugs) and coexisting haemodynamic status. Thus cardiac monitoring is no substitute for the skilled bedside assessment of the patient.

Reasons for the procedure

⌘   To identify and diagnose underlying cardiac disorders
⌘   To monitor effectiveness of treatment
⌘   To give a baseline of the patient's heart rhythm before treatment
⌘   To monitor the patient who is likely to have arrhythmias – for example, acute coronary syndromes, post-surgery, drug overdoses, electrical injuries and hypothermia
⌘   To monitor for cardiac ischaemia and coronary artery occlusion.

Pre-procedure

Equipment required

⌘   Disposable chest electrodes x 3
⌘   Monitor cable
⌘   Cardiac monitor (in working order) with recording facilities conventionally set at 25 mm per second

✖ Hair clippers for removing chest hairs if needed
✖ Dry gauze to remove any loose, dry skin
✖ Alcohol wipes.

Specific patient preparation required

✖ Inform the patient about the requirement and nature of cardiac monitoring (Thompson et al, 1986; Jowett, 1997; Squires and Ciecior, 2001)
✖ Identify positioning of chest electrodes (*Figure 5.1*).

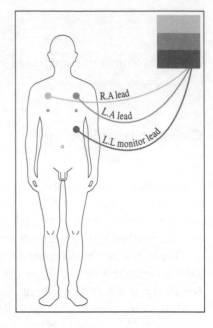

Figure 5.1: Three-electrode positioning system

During the procedure

✖ Clean the skin with alcohol wipes to ensure good contact
✖ Attach electrodes as in *Figure 5.1*
✖ Attach monitor cables to electrodes and the monitor
✖ Switch cardiac monitor on and set to lead II (Cooke and Metcalfe, 2000)
✖ The best possible trace should be attained. This includes a large enough waveform to see each component of the PQRST complex (*Figure 5.2*) and a clear, well-defined tracing that travels horizontally across the screen.
If the cardiac trace is poor, the nurse should troubleshoot for possible problems (*Box 5.4*).

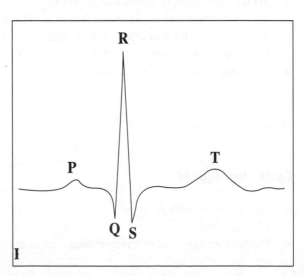

Figure 5.2: PQRST wave complex. P wave represents atrial depolarization; QRS wave represents ventricular depolarization; T wave represents ventricular repolarization

---

Box 5.4: Troubleshooting for cardiac trace abnormalities

Flat line trace	Ascertain that the monitor is in working order, that the correct monitoring leads have been selected, that the electrocardiogram gain is set correctly and that the electrodes are connected
Interference and artefacts	Ensure secure electrode contact and that electrodes are placed over bone rather than muscle. Keep the patient warm and note if any infusion pumps may be contributing to interference; if so, switch on the filter to eliminate background noise
Wandering baseline	The height of the QRS complexes vary in response to chest movement and the patient's position. In this instance the electrodes should be changed or a different monitoring lead selected

From Cooke and Metcalfe (2000); Jevon (2000)

Post-procedure

✿ Assess the cardiac trace (*Box 5.5*)

Box 5.5: Principles for assessing cardiac tracing

Analysis of cardiac rhythm requires an assessment of the PQRS and T waveforms. A systematic method of assessment includes the following:

✿ Rates of the P wave and the QRS complexes (they may not be the same)
✿ Regularity of the P wave and QRS complex
✿ Shape and size of the P wave and QRS complex and T wave
✿ Shape of the ST segment

✿ Report findings
✿ If abnormalities are present, perform a 12-lead ECG (see 'Recording a 12-lead ECG')
✿ Record findings in the patient's notes and inform medical staff as necessary
✿ Inform patient how attachment to continuous cardiac monitoring may affect their self-care abilities
✿ Check electrodes for any allergic reaction.

Student skill laboratory activity

✤ Identify the equipment you would require to set up cardiac monitoring

✤ Demonstrate the positioning of the electrodes on a manikin

✤ Consider some of the disorders that may require such an intervention.

Cardioversion

Cardioversion suspends an arrhythmia by simultaneously depolarizing most of the myocardium by delivering a synchronized electrical impulse, timed to begin at a particular phase in the heart's conduction cycle. The defibrillator senses the patient's conduction cycle and will automatically deliver the electrical current during the QRS complex.

The advantage of delivering a synchronized electrical current is to time the electrical discharge onto the R wave, thus avoiding the relative vulnerable period (*Figure 5.3*), during which the risk of inducing ventricular fibrillation (VF)/ventricular tachycardia (VT) is greatest. Riley (1997) provides an illustration to this effect. Synchronization should be used in all arrhythmias that are refractory to medical treatment and cause hypotension, cardiac failure or acute ischaemia, aside from VF and rapid VT (ventricular flutter) (Gordon, 1997).

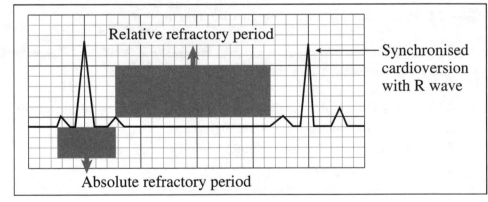

Figure 5.3: ECG showing absolute refractory and relative refractory periods

Reasons for the procedure

✤ To correct conduction disturbances
✤ To improve the effectiveness of the heart.

Pre-procedure

Equipment required

- ⌘ Defibrillator capable of providing a synchronized electrical current
- ⌘ Defibrillator gel pads
- ⌘ Continuous ECG monitor
- ⌘ Full resuscitation facilities with emergency drugs
- ⌘ Medications as requested by the anaesthetist.

Specific patient preparation required

- ⌘ Patient may be fasted for 6 hours before the procedure to prevent aspiration during sedation and anaesthesia
- ⌘ The patient's medication relevant to cardioversion should be reviewed. Digoxin levels should be checked as digoxin toxicity may increase the risk to induce VF/VT. Patients with atrial fibrillation who are treated with warfarin should have their INR/activated partial thromboplastin time (APTT) checked. The INR level should be maintained between 2.5–3.5 because of the risk of developing thromboembolism following cardioversion
- ⌘ A patent intravenous line should be available to administer sedation, anaesthesia and for emergency access
- ⌘ It may be necessary to shave the patient's chest if very hirsute to increase contact between the paddles and the patient's chest
- ⌘ Nitroglycerin patches should be removed from the patient's skin if used, as they may cause localized explosion triggered by electrical sparking
- ⌘ A 12-lead ECG recording should be obtained to record the patient's pre-cardioversion heart rhythm
- ⌘ Continuous ECG monitoring is essential to monitor the patient's heart rhythm during and after the procedure
- ⌘ Intranasal or facemask oxygen should be administered for at least 5 minutes before the procedure and should be monitored to achieve oxygen saturation of above 95%.

During the procedure

- ⌘ Select the lead position to obtain the best positive QRS complexes as the synchronization will sense the QRS complex
- ⌘ Pre-check for synchronization by selecting the synchronize button on the defibrillator when the patient is attached to the defibrillator monitor
- ⌘ Ensure that synchronization is achieved on 100% of QRS complexes. Changing the lead selection and increasing the amplitude on the defibrillator monitor may be necessary until 100% synchronization is achieved

⌘ Apply the defibrillator pad to the patient's chest to decrease thoracic impedance
⌘ Administer the prescribed sedation or anaesthesia (the anaesthetist)
⌘ Apply firm pressure to the paddles onto the patient's chest (see paddle position as in defibrillation procedure)
⌘ Recheck for synchronization
⌘ Check for safety (see 'Emergency defibrillation'). Shout all present to 'stand clear'
⌘ Deliver synchronized electrical current by holding down the discharge until electrical current has been delivered
⌘ It may take a few seconds before the defibrillator delivers the electrical current because it can only fire on the synchronized R wave. It is important that the pressure is applied continuously until the shock is delivered
⌘ Assess the patient's heart rhythm to check for cardioversion to sinus rhythm. The patient may develop transient junctional rhythm before reverting to sinus rhythm
⌘ Additional delivery of electrical current may be necessary and should be administered before the sedation wears off
⌘ Remove gel pads.

Post-procedure

⌘ The patient's airway should be cared for until full consciousness has returned. He/she may need to be positioned to ensure airway protection
⌘ Remain with the patient until vital signs, oxygen saturation and ECG are stable and the patient can maintain his/her airway safely
⌘ Monitor the patient's continuous ECG for several hours to detect for presence of arrhythmias
⌘ Obtain a 12-lead ECG to compare with pre-cardioversion ECG and confirm sinus rhythm
⌘ The outcome of the procedure, drugs administered and the cardioversion settings should be documented
⌘ Apply a cold, wet washcloth to the paddle sites to provide comfort and help reduce skin irritation
⌘ Report muscle soreness as increased levels of creatine phosphokinase, lactate dehydrogenase and aspartate aminotransferase are common complications after cardioversion and may indicate damage to tissues in the chest wall
⌘ The defibrillator should then be stored (see 'Care of the defibrillator').

Emergency defibrillation

Defibrillation is the delivery of a high-energy, non-synchronized current to the heart for the emergency treatment of ventricular fibrillation (VF) and pulseless ventricular tachycardia (VT) (Gordon, 1997). The defibrillator produces a direct current discharge, which travels between two electrodes (handheld paddles or adhesive patches) applied to the chest wall.

The electrical current depolarizes the myocardium through which it travels, hence suspending the chaotic impulses of VF and disrupting the continuous re-entry circuits often associated with tachyarrhythmia such as VT. It is imperative that a diagnosis of VF or pulseless VT is confirmed from the ECG monitor or from the defibrillator paddle before defibrillation is performed (Resuscitation Council UK, 2002).

Reasons for the procedure

❋ To terminate VF and pulseless VT and allow the restoration of normal conduction
❋ To prevent neurological damage and promote complete neurological recovery.

Pre-procedure

Equipment required

❋ Defibrillator
❋ Defibrillator gel pads
❋ Continuous ECG monitor
❋ Full resuscitation facilities with emergency drugs.

Specific patient preparation required

❋ Basic life support if necessary
❋ Continuous ECG monitoring should be established
❋ It is essential to avoid placing the ECG electrodes near the defibrillator gel pads to prevent burn
❋ Consider factors that may affect successful defibrillation (*Box 5.6*)

Box 5.6. Factors that may affect successful defibrillation

❋ The amount of current passing through the heart is determined by both the energy level selected and the transthoracic impedance

❋ The thoracic impedance is influenced by:

— the size of the electrode or paddle

— the paddle–skin interface material

— number and time interval of previous shock

— phase of ventilation

— distance between the electrodes

— paddle pressure

From White *et al* (2002)

✵ Applying firm pressure of approximately 10 kg in force to the paddles and discharging the current during the expiratory phase may reduce the transthoracic impedance (Resuscitation Council UK, 2002). Although it is quite difficult to judge how much pressure 10 kg in force would be, it is best to practise by pressing the hand on a bathroom scale to approximate the force required. Defibrillation should also be administered in close intervals as it reduces the impedance.

Safety

✵ Wipe away wet surroundings or materials or water from the patient's chest, as they are good conductors that attract electrical current and cause electrical burns
✵ Ensure that no part of any person comes into direct or indirect contact with the patient to prevent electrocution
✵ The defibrillator operator is responsible for ensuring that all persons are to stand clear by shouting 'stand clear' and checking that they have done so before discharging the electrical current
✵ Ensure that high-flow oxygen is not passing across the zone of defibrillation as spontaneous combustion may result.

During the procedure

1. Confirm cardiac arrest — check for signs of circulation for 10 seconds
2. Switch on equipment
3. Confirm VF/pulseless VT from ECG monitor or paddles
4. Place defibrillator gel pads on patient's chest. For the apex anterior position place one pad below the right clavicle and one over the cardiac apex (between the left fifth intercostal space in the anterior axillary line) (*Figure 5.4*). For the apex posterior position, place one paddle over the cardiac apex and the posterior paddle below the right scapula to the right of the spine (*Figure 5.5*)

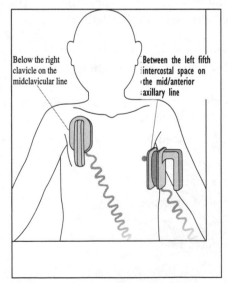

Figure 5.4: Apex anterior position

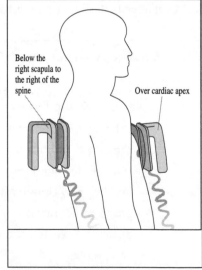

Figure 5.5: Apex posterior position

5. Place the defibrillator paddles firmly (using about 10 kg in force) on the gel pads
6. Select the correct energy level (either through the defibrillator or the paddles); start with 200 joules
7. Ensure high-flow oxygen is not crossing the zone of defibrillation
8. Press the charge button (either through the defibrillator or the paddles) only when the paddles are in contact with the patient's chest
9. Alert all present to 'stand clear' and perform visual check to ensure safety
10. Check monitor again to confirm VF/VT and discharge electrical current if VF/VT is presented.

If there is no response repeat the following

⌘ Maintain paddles on patient's chest
⌘ Ascertain rhythm on monitor (assistant to check pulse only if there is a change in the waveform on monitor)
⌘ If VF/pulseless VT persists, repeat steps 5–9 and deliver two more electrical currents. Ask an assistant to increase energy level to 200 joules, then to 360 joules if required
⌘ Defibrillation should not be interrupted for CPR unless the charging times are slow
⌘ After the third defibrillation, the paddles are to be replaced on the defibrillator. CPR should be continued if indicated for 1 minute, and the ALS algorithm (Resuscitation Council UK, 2002) should be followed.

Post-procedure

⌘ Switch defibrillator off
⌘ Clean paddles
⌘ Check and restock equipment
⌘ Return defibrillator and place on 'stand by'
⌘ Continue to treat and care for the patient accordingly.

Intra-aortic balloon pump

The intra-aortic balloon pump (IABP) procedure involves a polyurethane balloon being inserted through the femoral artery and placed in the descending aorta just distal to the left subclavian artery (Hebra and Kuhn, 1996). The IABP works by delivering more oxygen to the ischaemic myocardium. The IABP is triggered and timed to inflate the balloon at the beginning of diastole, hence increasing the pressure in the aorta. This rise in pressure forces blood into the coronary arteries, thus improving coronary perfusion. As the balloon deflates at the end of diastole, just before systole, it pulls blood forward into the unfilled space that was otherwise occupied by the inflated balloon. This reduces afterload and makes it easier for the left ventricle to eject its contents (Stamatis and Spadoni, 1997). This reduces the workload of the heart and also reduces myocardial oxygen demand. The increase in coronary perfusion and the reduced myocardial workload and oxygen demand are valuable in patients with left ventricular failure.

Reasons for the procedure

❋ To restore equilibrium in the heart after medical treatment (including vasodilators, diuretics, thrombolytics and positive inotropes) has not been effective in providing the balance between myocardial oxygen supply and demand (Stamatis and Spadoni, 1997).

Pre-procedure

Equipment required

❋ IABP console
❋ Helium gas cylinder
❋ ECG leads and cable
❋ Pressure transducer and cable
❋ Inflatable pressure bag
❋ ABP catheter kit. A spare kit should also be available
❋ ECG electrodes
❋ 500 ml 0.9% normal saline injectable solution, with 5000 units of heparin on a pressure bag
❋ Sterile gowns, gloves, drapes
❋ Povidone iodine solution
❋ Lidocaine for local anaesthetic
❋ Sutures
❋ Syringes and needles
❋ Emergency crash trolley with resuscitation drugs and equipment
❋ IABP record and checklist.

Equipment preparation

❋ The operator should be familiar with the functioning of the equipment
❋ Prime the 0.9% normal saline with the 5000 units of heparin through the pressure bag
❋ Set up sterile pressure transducer and zero at correct level
❋ Plug IABP console into mains power
❋ Turn on IABP console, verify there is a good ECG signal
❋ Ensure helium gas cylinder is turned on and canister is full
❋ Ensure trigger mode is set
❋ Ensure initial inflation/deflation settings are at 0.

Specific patient preparation required

- Verify that the patient has received heparin, and ideally an actual clotting time of 180–200 seconds is achieved from the time of insertion. This is to prevent clots from forming surrounding the balloon
- The patient is to lie flat and the head slightly elevated if presence of orthopnoea
- The patient's legs and vascular supply are examined to assess and select a favoured site
- Connect the patient to the ECG cables of the IABP console. Select a monitor lead that provides the best R wave and QRS complex, as the IABP console will use this to sense and trigger the pump to inflate and deflate the balloon
- Obtain baseline recording of the patient's oxygen saturation, pulse, blood pressure and a 12-lead ECG
- Assist in the setting up of an arterial line either through a radial artery or through the central lumen of the IABP catheter. This is necessary as the arterial line waveform is synchronized for timing of inflation and deflation of the balloon
- Provide education to patient regarding purpose of IABP and the importance of keeping the affected leg straight.

Insertion procedure

- Assist in the insertion of catheter
- Prepare and drape the patient to provide a sterile field
- Provide gowns, caps and mask to ensure strictest asepsis during procedure
- Usually a trained physician would insert the balloon catheter
- When the catheter has been correctly placed, the balloon lumen connection tubing is then attached to the console and the counterpulsation is initiated
- Assist in the suturing of the catheter at the insertion site to prevent dislodgement of the catheter.

Post-procedure

- Place a sterile dressing over the insertion site, keeping the site clean and dry
- Assess the balloon waveform for appropriate inflation and deflation (Stamatis and Spadoni, 1997)
- Set the pump alarm values
- Obtain a tracing of the arterial line with the IABP augmentation of 1:2 to document optimal timing. Document this at least every 8 hours to ensure continuity of care
- Observe the insertion site for swelling that may indicate haematoma or for any bleeding
- Check pedal pulses distal to the insertion site every 15 minutes for an hour, then 30 minutes for the next hour and then every hour to ensure adequate circulation
- Monitor the left radial/brachial artery pulses to ensure that the catheter has not migrated to the left subclavian artery causing occlusion to the circulatory flow
- Educate the patient to limit movement and ask for assistance in relation to activities of living.

Intravenous cannulation

Cannulation is the insertion of a short, flexible, plastic tube into a vein of the forearm or hand. A hollow needle is used as an introducer. It is one of the most common invasive procedures undertaken by nurses.

Reasons for the procedure

- ⌘ To administer drugs
- ⌘ To manage hydration and electrolyte imbalance/correct dehydration
- ⌘ To transfuse blood or blood components.

Pre-procedure

Equipment required

- ⌘ An appropriately sized cannula. Generally, the smallest possible gauge of cannula should be used (Jackson, 1997; Davies, 1998), and this should be inserted into the largest available vein
- ⌘ A clean surface to place equipment on
- ⌘ Disposable gloves
- ⌘ Tourniquet
- ⌘ Alcohol swab
- ⌘ Gauze
- ⌘ A suitably sized ported or non-ported cannula (*Box 5.7*)

Box 5.7: Cannula selection	
14–16 gauge	Major trauma/surgery, epidurals, massive rapid fluid replacement
18 gauge	Routine blood transfusions, rapid infusion
20 gauge	Routine infusions, bolus drug administration
22 gauge	Small, fragile veins, for short-term access
24 gauge	Small, fragile veins

From Jackson (1997)

- ⌘ A sterile dressing, following hospital policy/protocol (Fox, 2000), preferably a moisture-permeable transparent dressing

⌘ Tape to secure cannula
⌘ Other equipment (depending on the reason for cannulation) can include an administration set, extension set or injection cap, Luer-Lok plug (Dougherty, 2000a)
⌘ Possibly local anaesthesia cream or gel
⌘ Razor or scissors to cut hair (with permission).

Specific patient preparation required

⌘ Ensure that skin is clean and unnecessary hair removed
⌘ To improve venous access, ensure that the vein of the extremity that is intended for cannulation is below the level of the heart, clearly exposed and well supported
⌘ If the patient requests and if advisable, apply/use local anaesthetic cream/gel 15–30 minutes before insertion of the cannnula.

During the procedure

⌘ Carefully select an appropriate vein. This is usually from a choice of the forearm (*Figure 5.6*) or of the hand (*Figure 5.7*) as they are located just beneath the skin in the superficial fascia (Dougherty, 1996). Lower limbs should be avoided as there is an increased risk of deep vein thrombosis (Jackson, 1997). The factors shown in *Box 5.8* should be considered in site selection
⌘ Apply a tourniquet approximately 100–105 mm above the insertion site
⌘ Gently tap the vein to encourage venous filling
⌘ Cleanse the insertion site with an alcohol-based skin preparation and allow to dry for 30–60 seconds to minimize cross-infection by staff (Dougherty, 1996; Jackson, 1997; Davies, 1998)
⌘ Remove the needle cover of the cannula, fold down the wings of the cannula and grip appropriately
⌘ Draw the skin around the vein taut with the non-dominant hand, which will act as an anchor and prevent the vein from rolling (Dougherty, 1996)

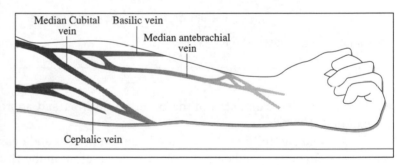

Figure 5.6: Veins of the forearm

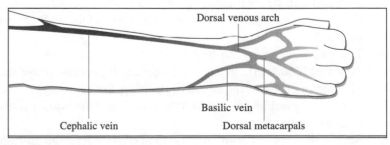

Figure 5.7: Veins of the hand

Box 5.8: Factors in site selection

The vein should	— be palpable
	— be easily visible
	— preferably have a large diameter and distal veins should be used first
	— preferably be on the non-dominant side of the patient
	— be on the opposite side to any surgical procedure
	— be straight
Avoid veins that	— have signs of inflammation, infection or bruising
	— are in areas of joint flexion
	— are close to arteries and deeper lying vessels
	— have been irritated from previous use
	— are antecubital fossa veins, as these are used for sampling venous blood
	— are thrombosed, sclerosed or fibrosed
	— are thin and fragile
	— are near a bony prominence
	— have undergone multiple punctures

From Dougherty (1996); Jackson (1997)

⌘ Ensure that the cannula is in the bevel up position and approach the vein on a low angle, for example 10–45°
⌘ Slowly and carefully push the cannula until it pierces and enters the vein
⌘ Successful entry is indicated by blood being present in the flashback chamber
⌘ Stop advancing the cannula briefly and reduce the angle of insertion to skin level
⌘ Ensure that the cannula is held securely and withdraw the inner needle and a secondary flashback of blood will be seen along the length of the cannula
⌘ Gradually insert the cannula into the vein while withdrawing the inner needle until it is fully inserted
⌘ The tourniquet can then be released
⌘ To avoid blood spillage press a finger on the vein or above the catheter tip, connect the Luer-Lok plug or appropriate equipment ensuring that it is tightly secured. The Luer-Lok plug can be removed by holding it between the thumb and the middle finger while pushing the needle forward with the index finger
⌘ Secure the cannula with tape and then cover with a moisture-permeable sterile dressing (Jackson, 1997).

Post-procedure

⌘ To verify the correct placement of the cannula, flush with sodium chloride 0.9%, but this may vary according to hospital policy/protocol

⌘ Document insertion of the cannula with appropriate care plan, ensuring all documentation is dated, timed and signed

⌘ The cannula site should be observed a minimum of once daily and when intravenous fluids are changed or intravenous medicines administered or according to hospital policy/protocol

⌘ Advise patient to maintain security and safety of the cannula

⌘ Monitor for complications that can occur as a consequence of cannulation (*Box 5.9*)

⌘ Dispose of sharps appropriately.

Box 5.9: Complications of cannulation	
Bacteraemia and sepsis	Fever, tachycardia leading to the life-threatening syndrome of septic shock (Davies, 1998)
Phlebitis and thrombophlebitis	Redness, tenderness and swelling around the site and the vein may be hard (Campbell, 1997)
Emboli	During insertion over the cannula the hollow must not be partly withdrawn from the cannula and reinserted as there is a risk of the needle cutting through the plastic cannula, and the cut part of the cannula may be carried away in the venous return to the heart (Campbell, 1997)
Vasovagal response	A drop in blood pressure and heart rate. Campbell (1997) suggests that those patients with a history of fainting may be advised to be recumbent instead of sitting up when cannulating
Infiltration and extravastion	Localized pain and swelling, blanching of the skin, coolness of the skin and leakage around the cannula. In the event of this happening, remove the cannula, elevate the limb to encourage lymphatic drainage. Certain medications can particularly irritate the vein and lead to localized tissue necrosis, e.g. fluids that are acid or alkaline, vasoconstricting, cytotoxic or hypertonic (Campbell, 1997; Davies, 1998)

Student skill laboratory activity
⌘ Assemble the equipment required to cannulate a patient
⌘ Identify veins on the forearm and hand on another student that could be cannulated
⌘ Practise cannulation on a manikin.

Intravenous infusion

Intravenous infusion is a method of administering fluids. This can include continuous infusion whereby a large volume of solution is administered over a prolonged period of time; an intermittent infusion where a relatively small amount of solution is administered over a short period of time; and a direct intermittent infusion, otherwise known as a bolus or direct injection, which is usually a drug injected into a vein via an infusion port.

Within this procedure the principles of infusing a large volume of solution or an intermittent amount will be addressed. This procedure does not discuss the administration of fluid using a pump. If it is anticipated that a pump can be used as a delivery device then manufacturer's guidelines must be followed.

The infusion of fluid can be referred to as 'fluid resuscitation' and can take the form of either colloid or crystalloid solutions (*Box 5.10*).

Box 5.10: Examples of crystalloids and colloids

Crystalloids	Colloids
Sodium chloride	Albumin, e.g. human albumin solution (HAS)
Sodium lactate (Hartmann's solution)	Hetastarch (Hespan), hexastarch (eloHAES) and pentastarch (HAES–steril, Hemohes and Pentaspan)
Glucose	Gelatin, e.g. Gelofusine, Haemaccel
Ringer's solution	
Dextrose saline	

From British Medical Association/Royal Pharmaceutical Society of Great Britain (BMA/RPSGB) (2004)

Reasons for the procedure

- ⌘ To replace lost fluid
- ⌘ Fluid resuscitation
- ⌘ Fluid challenge
- ⌘ Therapeutic use
- ⌘ Administer medication
- ⌘ Maintain hydration.

Pre-procedure

Equipment required

⌘ Tray to carry equipment
⌘ Prescription of the fluid to be infused therapy
⌘ Venous cannula *in situ* or equipment required for insertion of venous cannula (see 'Intravenous cannulation')
⌘ Fluid to infuse — this may come in a bag or in a rigid bottle
⌘ Drip/infusion stand
⌘ Appropriate giving set
⌘ Air inlet (if a rigid bottle is used)
⌘ Gloves
⌘ Gauze/sterile absorbent material
⌘ Tape (check for allergy).

Specific patient preparation required

⌘ The patient will have to be cannulated before commencement of intravenous therapy, and this should be checked for patency.

During the procedure

⌘ Assemble equipment in the tray
⌘ Check prescription chart with patient details (nameband and patient notes)
⌘ Check intravenous fluid as per local policy (observe that packaging is intact, note the expiry date, batch number and note for abnormalities within the fluid, such as foreign objects or clouding of the infusion therapy)
⌘ Take all items to the patient
⌘ Remove any outside packaging and hang the infusion bag on a drip stand. Remove packaging from the appropriate giving set and ensure that the roller clamp is closed (this is usually down). This prevents fluid flowing through, and therefore the risk of air bubbles is minimized (Dougherty, 2000b)
⌘ Remove the protective cover from around the infusion port – this can be done by twisting it off. This part of the infusion is now considered sterile
⌘ Expose the sterile spike of the giving set and fully insert the spike into the infusion port, being careful to maintain the sterility of both
⌘ If the solution to be infused is in a bottle then an air inlet should also be inserted, which is often identified on the top of the container
⌘ Squeeze the chamber until it is half way full

⌘ Hold the end that will be connected to the patient above the bag and partially open the roller clamp (this is usually mid-way) so that the giving set is 'primed'
⌘ Turn the roller clamp off. Put gloves on and remove the cap of the cannula
⌘ Remove the protective cap from the connector part of the giving set without contaminating it
⌘ Lock the end connector part of the giving set to the cannula, ensuring that this is screwed in firmly
⌘ To prevent complications such as kinking and pulling, the tubing should then be taped in an upwards direction using appropriate dressings
⌘ Commence the infusion by opening the roller clamp and adjust the flow rate as prescribed (ensuring manufacturer's guidance on drops/millilitre).

Post-procedure

⌘ Document all the information on the infusion chart/prescription chart
⌘ Enter amount of solution and type on the fluid balance chart
⌘ Ensure that the limb is adequately supported and advise patient how positioning could affect the infusion rate
⌘ Change infusion set and label according to local policy/protocol
⌘ Observe for potential complications (*Box 5.11*).

Box 5.11: Potential complications of intravenous infusion

Extravasation	The inadvertent administration of vesicant drugs into the surrounding tissues, which can result in tissue damage. Redness can present later alongside blistering, tissue necrosis and ulceration, burning or stinging pain, change in quality of infusion, leakage at the site and swelling (Dougherty, 2002)
Fluid overload	May result in pulmonary oedema, heart failure, arrhythmias and electrolyte imbalance
Infection	Redness and inflammation may be indicative, as well as a high temperature and raised pulse rate. Minimize interruption or disconnection of infusion (Fox, 2000)
Trauma	Perforation of the vein

Student skill laboratory activity

⌘ Assemble all the equipment required for setting up an infusion

⌘ Set up an infusion

⌘ Practise calculating flow rates for given volumes and given times as set by the instructor (Lapham and Agar, 1995).

Non-invasive temporary pacemaker

Non-invasive temporary pacemakers are used in emergency situations for temporary conduction disturbances. An electrical current is passed from an external pulse generator via a conducting cable and externally applied self-adhesive electrodes through the chest wall and heart.

Reasons for the procedure

⌘ To sustain the patient's rhythm until the conduction system returns to normal function or when a more definitive treatment is established (Corona, 1999)
⌘ To treat atropine-resistant symptomatic bradycardia or for asystole unresponsive to pharmacologic interventions (Keenan, 1995)
⌘ To terminate arrhythmias
⌘ When invasive pacing is contraindicated.

Pre-procedure

Equipment required

⌘ ECG monitor
⌘ Defibrillator with pacing capability
⌘ Transcutaneous electrodes
⌘ Emergency trolley with resuscitation medication and equipment
⌘ Oxygen.

Specific patient preparation required

⌘ Clip patient's hair if necessary to ensure good contact between the electrodes and patient's skin
⌘ Warn patient of discomfort caused by cutaneous nerve stimulation (tingling, stinging, pinching and burning) and skeletal muscle contraction (tapping, twitching).

During the procedure

⌘ Sedation may be prescribed if time permits
⌘ Connect the ECG monitoring electrodes to monitor the patient's ECG
⌘ Adjust the gain to obtain a QRS with adequate R wave height so that inappropriate discharge does not ensue

- Placement of pads. In the anterior-lateral placement (*Figure 5.8*), the lateral (apex) electrode is placed on the left anterior aspect of the torso, just lateral to the left nipple in the midaxillary line; this corresponds to the V6 electrode position. The anterior electrode is placed in the right subclavicular area lateral to the sternum

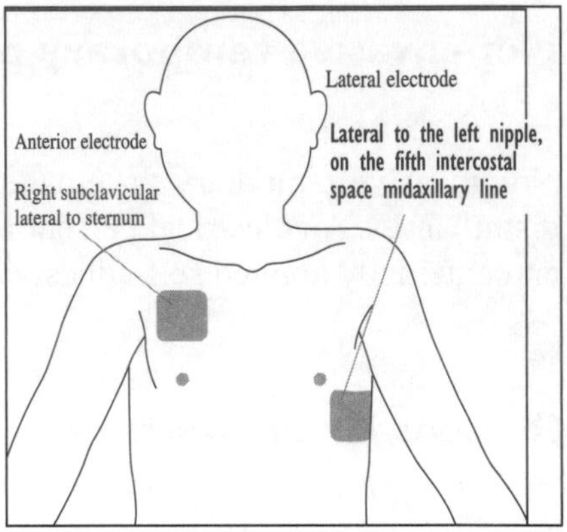

Figure 5.8: Anterior-lateral electrode placement

In anterior-posterior placement (*Figure 5.9*), the anterior electrode is placed on the left anterior aspect of the torso, halfway between the xiphoid process and left nipple at the apex of the heart. The upper edge of the electrode should be located below the nipple; this corresponds to the V2–V3 ECG electrode position. The posterior electrode is placed on the left posterior aspect of the torso beneath the scapula and lateral to the spine at the heart level. Placement of the electrodes over bony prominences such as the sternum, spine, or scapula should be avoided

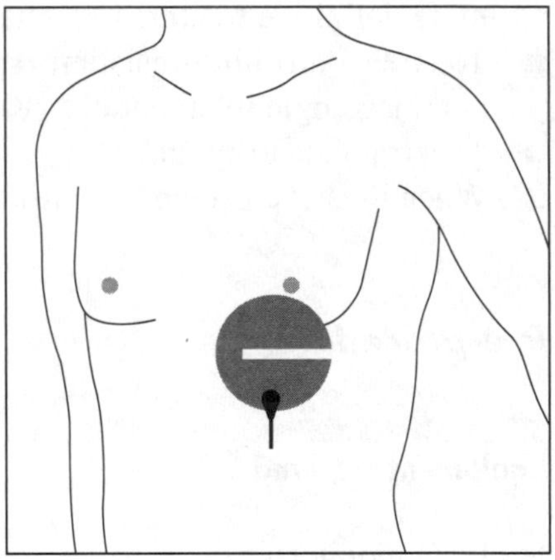

Figure 5.9: Anterior-posterior electrode placement

- Ensure that the electrical current is set to 0 before connecting the electrode cable to the monitor output cable
- Turn the pacing rate dial to 10 beats beyond the patient's intrinsic rhythm and observe for pacemaker spikes
- When spikes are observed, increase the electrical output until capture is obtained. Capture can be distinguished by each pacing spike being followed by a QRS complex
- When capture has been achieved, the electrical output is usually increased by 10% to maintain capture
- Select the pacing mode: demand or fixed as prescribed
- Document the paced rhythm, electrical output and rate.

Post-procedure

- Assess the patient's mental state or level of consciousness to evaluate pacemaker functioning
- Continue to monitor and record the patient's oxygen saturation, pulse and blood pressure
- Record a 12-lead ECG to evaluate pacemaker functioning

- ⌘ Ensure the pacing electrodes and cables are connected to maintain pacing function
- ⌘ Document date and time that pacing was initiated, pacing mode, rate and current required
- ⌘ Assist with activities of living as necessary
- ⌘ Prepare patient as required for further procedures
- ⌘ Manage treatment regimens accordingly.

Permanent pacemaker

A permanent pacemaker is an electronic device implanted under the skin of the patient's chest. It helps to maintain adequate heart rate and cardiac output in patients with conduction or impulse-initiation disorders. A pacemaker can be implanted through a thoracotomy, and the leads are usually introduced over a guidewire into the subclavian or jugular vein and threaded into place under fluoroscopy.

Pacemaker function

The pacemaker is capable of detecting the heart's intrinsic conduction; this function is referred to as the pacemaker's 'sensing' capability. The pacemaker is also able to produce an electrical impulse; this function of the pacemaker is referred to as the 'pacing' capability. The pacemaker consists of a pulse generator and one or two lead wires. The location of the pacer lead or leads will determine the heart chamber the device will pace and sense. The ability of a pacemaker to respond by either pacing or sensing is dependent on the mode of programmed operation.

The pacemaker is capable of triggering, inhibiting or dual response (trigger and inhibit). In a dual-response programme, the device senses an intrinsic beat in the atrium and it does not deliver an electrical charge to the ventricle if it senses an impulse in the ventricle within a pre-set time interval — referred to as the pacemaker's inhibitory response. If, however, the pre-set interval elapses without an intrinsic ventricular impulse, the pacemaker does deliver an impulse, called a triggered response.

The pacemaker can also be programmed to respond to the patient's activity level and minute ventilations. In this way, it can mimic the heart's natural function of increasing and decreasing heart rate to meet the body's needs (*Box 5.12*).

Box 5.12: Pacemaker codes			
Chamber paced	**Chamber sensed**	**Response to sensing**	**Programmability**
0: none	0: none	0: none	0: none
A: atrium programme	A: atrium	T: trigger	P: simple
V: ventricle	V: ventricle	I: inhibit	R: rate modulation
D: atrium and ventricle	D: atrium and ventricle	D: trigger and inhibitory	C: communication
			M: multi-programme

Leads are secured to the endocardium or sutured to the epicardium of the right atrium, right ventricle or both. Single-chamber pacemakers typically last 6–12 years; dual-chamber pacemakers last 4–8 years; and rate-responsive pacemakers last <4 years (Hasemeier, 1996).

Reasons for the procedure

⌘ Failure of the heart's conduction system to either initiate or conduct an intrinsic electrical impulse at a rate adequate to maintain effective perfusion (Corona, 1999)
⌘ Tachyarrhythmia when the heart rate is too fast to produce an effective ventricular contraction and cardiac output.

Pre-procedure

Equipment required

⌘ Antiseptic solution
⌘ Transvenous pacing catheter
⌘ Pacemaker generator with battery and cable (check patient's allergy or sensitivity to nickel or chromium, as a pulse generator coated with titanium would be used instead of stainless steel)
⌘ Introducer kit
⌘ Lidocaine (local anaesthetic)
⌘ Two 5 ml syringes with 22- and 25-gauge needles
⌘ Sterile gown, gloves, mask
⌘ ECG
⌘ Emergency trolley
⌘ Alligator clamps
⌘ Defibrillator
⌘ External pacer.

Prepare the external temporary generator by

⌘ Inserting a new battery
⌘ Turning the mA to 6
⌘ Turning the rate control to ten beats above the patient's baseline rate
⌘ Turning the sensitivity dial fully clockwise. The rate set above the patient's rate will suppress the patient's natural pacemaker.

Insertion sites

⌘ Left subclavian (mostly used), femoral vein, brachial vein
⌘ Internal jugular (lower incidence of pneumothorax).

Specific patient preparation required

⌘ The patient should be kept nil by mouth for at least 4–6 hours before implantation to prevent aspiration during sedation and anaesthesia

⌘ Assess mental status before, during and after the procedure to ascertain effectiveness of cardiac output and proper functioning of the implanted pacemaker

⌘ Obtain and record patient's respiratory rate and oxygen saturation for comparison during and after the procedure

⌘ Document apical and bilateral radial and pedal pulses and blood pressure to determine effectiveness of the pacemaker by comparing baseline value with post-implantation value

⌘ Record a 12-lead ECG for post-implantation evaluation

⌘ An intravenous line will be inserted to infuse fluids, a sedative and for emergency drugs access if needed

⌘ Prepare the patient's upper chest and abdomen as appropriate

⌘ Clean the side of the neck with antiseptic solution.

During the procedure

⌘ This is a medical procedure and the role of the nurse is to support the patient and assist the medical staff

⌘ Check that the patient has a patent IV, and that the defibrillator, emergency crash trolley and appropriate medications are available

⌘ Obtain vital signs and ECG rhythm strip before insertion. Connect to 12-lead ECG and continuously monitor before, during and after procedure

⌘ Prepare patient according to central line insertion procedure

⌘ Assist in the administration of lidocaine to the insertion area for local anaesthesia

⌘ Connect the alligator clamp: one end to the V1 ECG lead and the other to the distal or negative electrode wire of the pacemaker catheter. This electrode serves as an exploratory intracavity lead and the resulting ECG waveform helps to confirm electrode position

⌘ Monitor patient's vital signs and ECG while physician inserts pacing electrode.

Post-procedure

Observation

The nurse caring for the patient with an inserted permanent pacemaker needs to observe for the patient's oxygen saturation level, pulse rate and blood pressure. This should be done more frequently at the beginning, such as every 15 minutes for 1 hour, half-hourly for 1 hour and then hourly for

4 hours. It is essential that the patient's heart rate and blood pressure are monitored to ensure that the permanent pacemaker is producing an effective cardiac output. Observing the patient's mental status such as incidence of confusion or reduced level of consciousness may correlate with a reduced cardiac output.

ECG analysis

⌘ A post-pacemaker implant 12-lead ECG must be undertaken and compared with the pre-pacemaker implant 12-lead ECG. Further ECG monitoring should also be provided. The nurse should observe for any ischaemic or hyperacute changes and for arrhythmias
⌘ Any sign of loss of capture or failure to pace should be reported (Reynolds and Apple, 2001)
⌘ If the patient requires defibrillation, the paddle should be kept 7.5 cm away from the pulse generator
⌘ The nurse should also assess the insertion site for bleeding or infection
⌘ The patient's range of motion on the affected side should be limited
⌘ The nurse should also observe for other complications, such as perforations, haemorrhage, pneumothorax, haemothorax and tamponade.

Patient education

The patient should be taught about the need to:

⌘ Inspect the insertion site for evidence of infection
⌘ Report light-headedness, syncope (fainting), fever or skin discoloration
⌘ Avoid high-output electrical generators, contact sports and tight clothing
⌘ Inform healthcare providers about the present pacemaker.

Pericardiocentesis

Pericardiocentesis involves the use of a needle to aspirate fluid from the membrane that surrounds the heart (Fagan and Chan, 1999). Since the development of 2-dimensional echocardiography to guide the position of the needle, serious complications such as injury to the liver, myocardium, coronary arteries and lungs have been greatly reduced. Because 2-dimensional echocardiography permits direct visualization of cardiac structures and the adjacent vital organs, the procedure is now performed with minimal risk.

Reasons for the procedure

⌘ To remove fluid that is compressing the heart
⌘ For diagnostic purposes.

Pre-procedure

Equipment required

- ⌘ 18- to 20-gauge cardiac needle or long central venous catheter with needle introducer
- ⌘ Three-way stopcock
- ⌘ Syringes (10, 20 and 50 ml)
- ⌘ Chlorhexidine and alcohol or povidone-iodine solution
- ⌘ Pre-labelled specimen collection tubes for pericardial fluid analysis and cultures
- ⌘ Small-gauge needle for local anaesthesia and 1 or 2% lidocaine (as prescribed)
- ⌘ Sterile gloves, mask, gown, dressing materials and gauze
- ⌘ Surgical blade (#11)
- ⌘ Multiple 16- to 18-gauge venous cannula
- ⌘ Sterile sodium chloride solution (for flushing catheter)
- ⌘ Emergency crash trolley
- ⌘ Sedating medications
- ⌘ Defibrillator with monitor.

Specific patient preparation required

- ⌘ A 2-dimensional echocardiography must be performed before the pericardiocentesis to assess the size of the effusion
- ⌘ Blood tests including full blood count, urea and electrolytes, group and match and clotting profile should have been undertaken before the procedure
- ⌘ Protamine (blood-clotting protein) should be administered to correct the clotting time, and heparin should be discontinued
- ⌘ A 12-lead ECG should be performed and the patient must be monitored by continuous ECG
- ⌘ An intravenous line with an ongoing infusion of normal saline or 5% dextrose.

During the procedure

- ⌘ This procedure is performed by a trained physician
- ⌘ Throughout the procedure, the patient's oxygen saturation, pulse, ECG and blood pressure must be monitored
- ⌘ Assist the patient in sitting upright with 30–45° head elevation. This would increase the pooling of fluid toward the inferior and anterior surface of the pericardium, thus maximizing fluid drainage
- ⌘ The physician will select a site that is closest to the pericardial space, avoiding vital structures, such as the internal mammary artery, lungs, myocardium, liver and vascular bundle at the inferior margin of each rib
- ⌘ The patient's hair surrounding the area is normally shaved

⌘ The area for the needle insertion is anesthetized with lidocaine (1–2%)

⌘ A small incision (approximately 5 mm) is made to decrease the resistance during needle insertion

⌘ The subcutaneous tissue would normally be separated with a mosquito-grasping forceps

⌘ Assist in the connection of the needle with a three-way stopcock

⌘ A syringe with 1% lidocaine may be connected to the three-way stopcock on the opposite side of the needle connection, to enhance anaesthesia when the needle is inserted

⌘ Assist in the connection of the syringe on the other side of the three-way stopcock. Attach a sterile ECG alligator clip to the metal part of the needle to facilitate correct needle positioning. The ECG alligator clip is then connected to an ECG monitor

⌘ The needle is inserted through the sub-xiphoid approach on the left side. Sometimes a fluoroscopy or 2-dimensional echocardiography may be used to assist in the procedure

⌘ Monitor the ECG for ST elevation. Inform the physician of ST elevation as the needle may be inserted into the myocardium

⌘ When the needle tip is inside the pericardial space, a soft floppy-tip guidewire is passed through the needle. The needle is then removed and a catheter is pushed through the guidewire

⌘ The guidewire is removed and a syringe with a three-way stopcock is connected to the needle. Pericardial fluid is then aspirated and required samples sent to the laboratory

⌘ After the procedure the needle is then removed

⌘ Place a dressing over the site.

Post-procedure

⌘ The patient's oxygen saturation, pulse, ECG and blood pressure are monitored and recorded as clinically indicated

⌘ Dispose of sharps as per local policy.

Recording an ECG

An ECG is an electrical recording of the heart and is used in the investigation of heart disease. An ECG may appear normal even in the presence of significant heart disease, and therefore a full assessment of the heart may require additional tests.

Reasons for the procedure

⌘ Monitor haemodynamic stability

⌘ Identify different types of heart disorders

⌘ Aid diagnosis of pain

- ⌘ Identify disorders of the coronary arteries
- ⌘ Monitor the effectiveness of medication
- ⌘ Reveal rhythm problems
- ⌘ Detect electrolyte abnormalities.

Pre-procedure

Equipment required

- ⌘ ECG machine
- ⌘ Alcohol wipes
- ⌘ Hair clippers
- ⌘ Tissues.

Specific patient preparation

- ⌘ Ensure that the ECG equipment is in good working order. The operator should be familiar with the operation of the equipment
- ⌘ The patient must be stripped to the waist to expose the chest
- ⌘ Ensure the patient is in a supine position
- ⌘ Clean limbs and chest electrode sites
- ⌘ If necessary, hairs may be clipped to ensure good contact between the skin and the electrode.

During the procedure

⌘ Apply the self-adhesive electrodes on the limbs and chest. Attach the limb electrodes on the palmar aspect of the hand and one on each ankle. The chest leads are placed as follows (*Figure 5.10*):

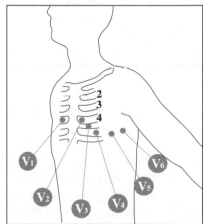

— V1 on the fourth intercostal space, right sternal edge
— V2 on the fourth intercostal space, left sternal edge
— V4 place before the third electrode. This is placed in the fifth intercostal space in the mid-clavicular line
— V3 placed half way between the second and fourth electrodes
— V5 lies on the fifth rib in the anterior axillary line
— V6 on an imaginary horizontal line with V5 in the midaxillary line

Figure 5.10: Chest leads

⌘ Attach the respective leads from the ECG machine to the electrodes, ensuring that the leads are connected correctly
⌘ Ask patient to relax and keep still
⌘ Check the calibration is set at the standard rate on the ECG machine at 10 mg/millivolt
⌘ Operate the ECG machine so that a 12-lead ECG is produced.

Post-procedure

⌘ After the recording, inform the patient that the procedure is complete. Remove the leads and electrodes
⌘ Label the ECG correctly with the patient's names, date, time and the hospital number
⌘ Inform medical staff that the ECG has been completed.

Student skill laboratory activity

⌘ Position electrodes on a manikin that can simulate an ECG recording
⌘ Record an ECG
⌘ Identify the normal PQRST wave complex
⌘ Calculate the heart rate from the ECG recording
⌘ Identify the rhythm.

Venepuncture

Venepuncture has been defined as the incision of a vein in order to obtain a specimen of blood (Anderson and Anderson, 1995). Venepuncture is a common procedure undertaken to aid diagnosis. The best veins are usually found at the elbow, in the antecubital fossa. These veins are easier to puncture because they can be anchored by pulling the skin tight over the vein, and they may be less painful than veins in the back of the hand or lower arm. For these reasons, this procedure will describe venepuncture from the antecubital fossa site only.

Reasons for the procedure

⌘ To identify the cause of an illness, such as infection, anaemia, allergies
⌘ To determine blood-clotting time, blood type for grouping and cross-matching and values of blood-cell type (Evans et al, 2003)
⌘ To determine levels of chemical substances within the blood.

Pre-procedure

Equipment required

- ⌘ Completed request form(s)
- ⌘ Clean tray
- ⌘ Non-sterile gloves and apron
- ⌘ Tourniquet
- ⌘ Alcohol wipes
- ⌘ Cotton wool balls or gauze swabs
- ⌘ Small, self-adhesive, sterile dressing (ensure patient is not allergic to adhesive)
- ⌘ Sharps container
- ⌘ Vacutainer with needle and vacuum sampling tubes or 21-gauge needle with syringes and appropriate sample tubes. Size of syringe will depend on amount of blood required for sample.

Specific patient preparation required

- ⌘ Ensure that the patient is sitting or lying down comfortably
- ⌘ Identify a suitable vein for venepuncture (usually antecubital fossa), ensuring that there are no intravenous infusions/transfusions *in situ*.

During the procedure

- ⌘ Support the chosen arm under the elbow with a pillow and position the arm straight and extended, palm uppermost (*Figure 5.11*). (To increase blood flow, the arm can be placed with the hand downwards towards the floor to encourage filling of the veins by gravity. The patient may also be asked to clench and unclench their hand to encourage arterial flow.)
- ⌘ Assemble equipment by twisting the needle clockwise onto the vacutainer or place the 21-gauge needle on to a suitably selected syringe and check for patency
- ⌘ Apply disposable gloves
- ⌘ Cleanse the skin and around the intended puncture site with an alcohol wipe for at least 30 seconds and allow to dry (Franklin, 1999)

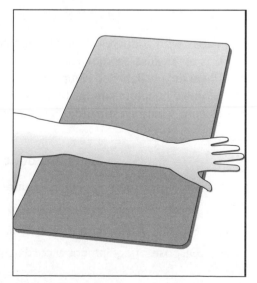

Figure 5.11: Arm supported

⌘ Label the blood bottles by the bedside to reduce risk of errors (British Committee for Standards in Haematology, 2003); crosscheck the patient's identification with the request form

⌘ Apply the tourniquet approximately 8–10 cm above the intended site around the upper arm and tighten it. It should not be applied for longer than 1 minute before collecting the blood specimen, as prolonged use will cause intravascular fluid to leak into the tissues and may affect the accuracy of the test

⌘ Palpate the vein to locate its position and its direction. Also note elasticity and depth of the vein. Visualization of the vein may be more difficult in obese patients, and palpation is a more accurate method of ascertaining condition of the vein than appearance

⌘ Holding the syringe and needle/vacuum container in the dominant hand, use the non-dominant hand to anchor the vein using the thumb to pull the skin tightly downwards. With the bevel of the needle uppermost and directly over the vein, insert the needle at an angle of about 45° through the skin and into the vein aligned along its direction, to approximately 2 mm depth into the lumen of the vein. Blood will appear in the syringe/vacuum sampling tube. Withdraw the required amount

⌘ If using a syringe, avoid pulling too vigorously on the plunger of the syringe as this may cause the vein to collapse. Remove needle and transfer the sample from the syringe into a suitable pre-labelled sample tube

⌘ Loosen the tourniquet, hold a gauze or cotton wool swab over the puncture site and gently withdraw the needle. Do not add pressure to the site until the needle is completely withdrawn, as this is more painful and may cause trauma to the wall of the vein

⌘ Continue to apply pressure on the puncture site until haemostasis occurs (approximately 2 minutes unless the patient is taking anticoagulants, which may extend this time) with the arm remaining extended as this may help to prevent bruising

⌘ Using a non-resheathe technique, dispose of sharps as per local policy

⌘ Apply a suitably sized adhesive dressing, ensuring that the patient is not allergic to the adhesive

⌘ Remove gloves.

Post-procedure

⌘ Tubes with additives should be gently inverted to mix the contents, but should not be shaken as this may cause haemolysis

⌘ Place the pre-labelled sample tubes with the correct request forms in the appropriate plastic bags

⌘ Monitor puncture site for bruising, haemorrhage, haematoma and infection

⌘ Record what investigations have been requested.

Student skill laboratory activity

⌘ Assemble the equipment required to undertake venepuncture

⌘ Locate the vein of the antecubital fossa on a colleague and on the manikin

⌘ Practice venepuncture on the manikin

⌘ Dispose of equipment accordingly.

Thrombolysis

Thrombolytic agents work by dissolving the fibrin network holding a thrombus together, causing it to break apart (Palatnik, 2000). This enables blood flow to be restored to the heart muscle, potentially salvaging damaged myocardium.

Currently four thrombolytic agents are licensed for use in the UK (National Institute for Clinical Excellence (NICE), 2002). These can be separated into two distinct groups:

⌘ *Streptokinase,* derived from streptococcal bacteria. Antibodies are produced after the first dose; as a consequence it can only be used once (BMA/RPSGB, 2004)
⌘ *Plasminogen activators,* produced using DNA recombinant technology (alteplase, reteplase, tenecteplase). These agents may be administered on more than one occasion, as antibodies are not produced after administration.

The efficacy of thrombolysis is directly related to the speed at which it is administered after symptom onset, with maximum benefit achieved within the first 2 hours (Boersma et al, 1996).

Reasons for the procedure

⌘ To dissolve a thrombus
⌘ Re-establish circulation
⌘ Minimize further complications.

Pre-procedure

Equipment required (dependent on the agent being administered)

⌘ Drug as prescribed
⌘ Infusion device
⌘ Intravenous fluid as prescribed
⌘ Giving set
⌘ Three-way stopcock
⌘ Syringes (various sizes)
⌘ Needles (various gauges)
⌘ Alcohol wipes
⌘ Sharps bin
⌘ Appropriate dressing.

Specific patient preparation required

✤ A 12-lead ECG showing evidence of ST elevation, post-myocardial infarction or new left-bundle branch block has been recorded and criteria for thrombolysis are satisfied

✤ The patient is attached to a cardiac monitor

✤ Bilateral blood pressures have been recorded, to exclude aortic dissection and hypertension

✤ A cannula has been inserted

✤ Bloods for urea and electrolytes, creatinine kinase, cholesterol, glucose and, if appropriate, troponin have been sent

✤ Exclude all absolute contraindications (*Box 5.13*) (Connaughton, 2002; Ghuran et al, 2003; Jowett and Thompson, 2003).

Box 5.13: Absolute and relative contraindications to thrombolysis

Absolute contraindications to thrombolysis	Active bleeding (not menstruation)
	Gastrointestinal bleed within the last month
	Suspected aortic dissection
	Major surgery within the last 3 weeks
	Intracranial neoplasm
	Cerebrovascular accident (CVA) within past 12 months/ previous CVA with permanent disability
Relative contraindications	Uncontrolled hypertension (blood pressure in excess of 180/100)
	Recent trauma (within past 4 weeks)
	Cerebrovascular surgery
	Traumatic cardiopulmonary resuscitation
	Anticoagulant therapy
	Aortic aneurysm
	Advanced liver disease
	Intracardiac thrombus
	Active peptic ulceration, varices
	Pregnancy
	Transient ischaemic attack within the past 3 months
	Diabetic retinopathy

From Connaughton (2002); Ghuran *et al* (2003); Jowett and Thompson (2003)

During the procedure

- ⌘ Assemble equipment and devices according to manufacturer's guidelines
- ⌘ Prepare medication as prescribed
- ⌘ Administer the drug as appropriate
- ⌘ Monitor for complications during the procedure (*Box 5.14*).

Box 5.14: Complications of thrombolytic therapy

Severe hypotension (most common with streptokinase) – should this occur, lay the patient flat, drop his/her head and stop the infusion if the reaction is severe. IV colloid therapy may be warranted (Connaughton, 2002)

Allergic reactions/anaphylaxis (most common with streptokinase) – stop the infusion. The patient may require treatment with IV hydrocortisone 100 mg, IV chlorpheniramine 100 mg. An alternate thrombolytic agent may be required (Connaughton, 2002)

Cerebral haemorrhage/cerebral vascular accident (CVA) (risk slightly elevated with alteplase and reteplase) – observe the patient for reduced consciousness/severe headache. Stop the infusion. Computed tomography scan will be required to confirm the diagnosis. Anticoagulant effect may be reversed with fresh frozen plasma (FFP) and IV protamine if heparin is given. Specialist neurology opinion may be required. CVA is thought to occur in 0.2–1% of cases (Jowett and Thompson, 2003)

Systemic haemorrhage – observe the patient for signs of bleeding and/or hypovolaemic shock. Treatment will depend on the site of the bleeding and will range from the application of direct pressure to the transfusion of FFP and blood. Strict observation of pacing wire and central line sites is required, and unnecessary line insertion should be avoided. Specialist advice from a surgeon/haematologist should be sought if necessary

---

Post-procedure

- ⌘ Perform an ECG 60–90 minutes after drug administration to assess response of re-perfusion therapy depending on local policy
- ⌘ Ensure documentation is completed, including the name and date of the drug given
- ⌘ Continue to monitor for complications
- ⌘ Dispose of equipment as per local policy.

References

Anderson K, Anderson L (1995) *Mosby's Pocket Dictionary of Nursing, Medicine and Professionals Allied to Medicine*. Times Mirror Publishing, London

Atterbury C (2001) Practical procedures for nurses: blood transfusion – part 1. *Nurs Times* **97**(2): 45–6

Boersma E, Maas A, Deckers J, Simoons M (1996) Early thrombolytic treatment in acute myocardial infarction: reappraisal of the golden hour. *Lancet* **348:** 771–5

Bradbury M, Cruickshank JP (2000) Blood transfusion: crucial steps in maintaining safe practice. *Br J Nurs* **9:** 134–8

British Committee for Standards in Haematology (2003) *Serious Hazards of Transfusion: Annual Report 2001–2002*. BCSH, Manchester

British Medical Association/Royal Pharmaceutical Society of Great Britain (2004) *British National Formulary*. BMA/RPSGB, London

Campbell J (1997) Intravenous cannulation: potential complications. *Prof Nurse* **12**(Suppl 8): S10–S13

Connaughton M (2002) *Evidence-based Coronary Care*. Elsevier Science, Edinburgh

Cooke F, Metcalfe H (2000) Cardiac monitoring – 2. *Nurs Times* **96**(25): 45–6

Copp J (2001a) Bone marrow aspiration and biopsy – 1. *Nurs Times* **97**(29): 45–6

Copp J (2001b) Bone marrow aspiration and biopsy – 2. *Nurs Times* **97**(31): 45–6

Copp J (2001c) Bone marrow aspiration and biopsy – 3. *Nurs Times* **97**(32): 43–4

Corona G (1999) Pacemakers: keeping the beat today. *RN* **62**(12): 50–6

Davies SR (1998) The role of nurses in intravenous cannulation. *Nurs Stand* **12**(17): 43-6

Dougherty L (1996) Intravenous cannulation. *Nurs Stand* **11**(2): 47–53

Dougherty L (2000a) Care of a peripheral intravenous cannula. *Nurs Times* **96**(5): 51–2

Dougherty L (2000b) Practical procedures for nurses: priming an infusion set – 1. *Nurs Times* **96**(6): 49–50

Dougherty L (2002) Delivery of intravenous therapy. *Nurs Stand* **16**(16): 45–52

Evans DMD, Evans C, Evans RA (2003) *Special Tests: The Procedure and Meaning of Common Hospital Tests*. 5th edn. Mosby, China

Fagan S, Chan KL (1999) Pericardiocentesis: blind no more! *Chest* **116**(2): 275–6

Fox N (2000) Managing the risks posed by intravenous therapy. *Nurs Times* **96**(30): 37–9

Franklin L (1999) Skin cleansing and infection control in peripheral venepuncture and cannulation. *Nurs Stand* **14**(4): 49–50

Ghuran A, Uren N, Nolan J (2003) *Emergency Cardiology: An Evidence-based Guide to Acute Cardiac Problems*. Oxford University Press, London

Gordon SPF (1997) Cardioversion and defibrillation. In: Thomson PL, ed. *Coronary Care Manual*. Churchill Livingstone, New York: 361–7

Hasemeier CS (1996) Permanent pacemaker. *Am J Nurs* **96**(2): 30–1

Hebra J, Kuhn M (1996) *Manual of Critical Care Nursing: Critical Care Fact Finder*. Little, Brown and Company, Boston.

Jackson A (1997) Performing peripheral intravenous cannulation. *Prof Nurse* **13:** 21–5

Jevon P (2000) Cardiac monitoring. *Nurs Times* **96**(23): 43–4

Jowett NI (1997) *Cardiovascular Monitoring*. Whurr Publishers, London

Jowett N, Thompson D (2003) *Comprehensive Coronary Care*. 3rd edn. Elsevier Science, Edinburgh

Keenan J (1995) Temporary cardiac pacing. *Nurs Stand* **9**(20): 50–1

Loach J, Thomson NB (1987) *Haemodynamic Monitoring*. Lippincott, Philadelphia

Marieb EN (2004) *Human Anatomy and Physiology*. 6th edn. Pearsons Benjamin Cummings, San Francisco

Mawer RJ, Bigham R, Macnab JA (1999) Vascular access. In: Macnab A, Macrae D, Henning R, eds. *Care of the Critically Ill Child*. Churchill Livingstone, London

National Institute for Clinical Excellence (2002) *Drugs for Early Thrombolysis in the Treatment of Acute Myocardial Infarction*. The Stationery Office, London

Palatnik A (2000) Acute coronary syndrome: new advances and practices. *Dimens Crit Care Nurs* **19**(5): 22–6

Perry AG, Potter PA (1994) *Clinical Nursing Skills and Techniques*. Mosby, St Louis

Resuscitation Council UK (2002) *Advanced Life Support Provider Manual*. 4th edn. Resuscitation Council UK, London

Reynolds J, Apple S (2001) A systematic approach to pacemaker assessment. *Advanced Practice in Acute and Critical Care* **12**(1): 114–26

Riley MC (1997) Elective cardioversion: who, when, and how. *RN* **60**(5): 27–9

Royal College of Nursing (2004) *Right Blood, Right Patient, Right Time: RCN Guidance for Improving Transfusion Practice*. RCN, London

Squires A, Ciecior D (2001) Teaching telemetry. *Nurs Manage* **32**: 43–6

Srejic U, Wenker OC (2003) A-line or intra-arterial catheters. *Internet Journal of Health* **3**(1). www.ispub.com/ostia/index.php?xmlFilePath=journals/ijh/vol3n1/aline.xml (last accessed 3 June 2005)

Stamatis SJ, Spadoni SM (1997) Getting to the heart of IABP therapy. *RN* **60**(1): 38–44

Stansby G, Smout J, Chalmers R, Lintott P (2003) MRSA infected pseudoaneurysms of the radial artery. *Surgeon* **1**: 108–10

Thompson D, Bailey S, Webster R (1986) Patients' views on cardiac monitoring. *Nurs Times* **82**(25): 54–5

Tremayne P (2003) Case 20 'Blood transfusion'. In: Parboteeah S, Tremayne P. *Client Profile in Nursing: Adult and The Elderly 2*. Greenwich Medical Media, London

Trewhitt KG (2001) Bone marrow aspiration, biopsy collection and interpretation. *Oncol Nurs Forum* **28**(9): 1409–17

Way C (2000) Monitoring physiological signs. In: Williams C, Asquith J, eds. *Paediatric Intensive Care Nursing*. Churchill Livisgtone, London

White RD, Blackwell TH, Russell JK (2002) The influence of transthoracic impedance on defibrillation, resuscitation and survival in out-of-hospital cardiac arrest treated by basic life support providers with an impedance-compensated biphasic waveform automatic external defibrillator. *Ann Emerg Med* **40**(4 Pt 2): S95–S96

Further reading

Anonymous (2002) Common cardiac arrhymias. *Emerg Nurse* **10**: 29–40

Buckley R (1999) Keep it legal. *Nurs Times* **95**(6): 75–9

Campbell H, Carrington M, Limber C (1999) A practical guide to venepuncture and management of complications. *Br J Nurs* **8**(7): 426–31

Cooke F (2000) Cardiac monitoring – 1. *Nurs Times* **96**(23): 45–6

Cooke F (2000) Cardiac monitoring – 2. *Nurs Times* **96**(25): 45–6

Cooke F, Metcalfe H (2000) Cardiac monitoring – 1. *Nurs Times* **96**(23): 45–6

Department of Health (2000) *The National Service Framework for CHD*. The Stationery Office, London

Docherty B, Roe J (2001) Cardiac arrhythmias: recognition and care. *Prof Nurse* **16:** 1492–6

Dougherty L (1996) Intravenous cannulation. *Nurs Stand* **11**(2): 47–51

Dougherty L (2000) Practical procedures for nurses: priming an infusion set – 2. *Nurs Times* **96**(7): 51–2

Drew BJ (2002) Celebrating the 100th birthday of the electrocardiogram: lessons learned form research in cardiac monitoring. *Am J Crit Care* **11:** 376–89

Dunn DL, Gregory JJ (1989) Non invasive temporary pacing: experience in community hospital. *Heart Lung* **18:** 23–8

Edwards S (2000) Fluid overload and monitoring indices. *Prof Nurse* **15:** 568–72

Fibrinolytic Therapy Trialists Collaborative Group (1994) Indications for fibrinolytic therapy in suspected acute myocardial infarction: collaborative overview of early mortality and major morbidity results from all randomised trials of over 1000 patients. *Lancet* **343:** 311–22

Gamrath B, Del Monte L, Richards K (1998) Non-invasive pacing: what you should know. *J Emerg Nurs* **24**(3): 223–33

Golding MA, Palmer GD, Fleming GJ (2002) Preference for venepuncture site: should the patient be consulted? *Dent Update* **29**(5): 239–43

Grech E, Ramsdale D (2003) Acute coronary syndrome: ST segment myocardial infarction. *Br Med J* **326:** 1379–81

Hand H (2001) The use of intravenous therapy. *Nurs Stand* **15**(43): 47–52

Hand H (2002) Common cardiac arrhythmias. *Nurs Stand* **16**(28): 43–52

Hansen HC, Harboe H, Drenck NE (1989) Bruising after venepuncture [Article in Danish]. *Ugeskr Laeger* **151**(10): 626–7

Heath S, Bain R, Andrews A, Chida S, Kitchen S, Walters M (2003) Nurse initiated thrombolysis in the emergency department: safe, accurate, and faster than fast track. *Emergency Med J* **20:** 418–20

Hebra JD (1994) The nurse's role in continuous dysrhythmia monitoring. *AACN Clin Issues Crit Care Nurs* **5:** 178–85

Hoit B (2002) Management of effusive and constrictive pericardial heart disease. *Circulation* **105**(25): 2939–42

Hutchisson B, Cossey S, Wheeler R (2003) Basic electrocardiogram interpretation for perioperative nurses. *AORN J* **78**(4): 572–90

Hyde L (2002) Legal and professional aspects of intravenous therapy. *Nurs Stand* **16**(26): 39–42

Jacobsen C (2003) Bedside cardiac monitoring. *Crit Care Nurse* **23:** 71–4

Lapham R, Agar H (1995) *Drug Calculations for Nurses: A Step by Step Approach*. Arnold, London

McConnell E (2001) Applying cardiac monitor electrodes. *Nursing* **31**(8): 17

McIntosh N (2000) Implementing clinical education for phlebotomists. *Nurs Stand* **15**(1): 43–6

Metcalfe H (2000) Recording a 12-lead electrocardiogram, part 1. *Nurs Times* **96**(19): 43–4

Metcalfe H (2000) Recording a 12-lead electrocardiogram, part 2. *Nurs Times* **96**(21): 45–6

Metcalfe H (2000) Recording a 12-lead electrocardiogram, part 3. *Nurs Times* **96**(22): 45–6

Mond GH (1997) Cardiac pacemakers. In: Thomson PL, ed. *Coronary Care Manual*. Churchill Livingstone, New York, 367–72

Navas S (2003) Atrial fibrillation: part 2. *Nurs Stand* **17**(38): 47–54

Oldroyd K (2000) Identifying failure to achieve complete (Timi III) reperfusion following thrombolytic treatment: how to do it, when to do it and why it is worth doing. *Heart* **83:** 113–15

Persons CB (1986) External cardiac pacing in the emergency department. *J Emerg Nurs* **12:** 348–52

Pryke S (2004) Advantages and disadvantages of colloid and crystalloid fluids. *Nurs Times* **100**(10): 32–3

Quasim A, Malpass K, O'Gorman D, Heber M (2002) Safety and efficacy of nurse-initiated thrombolysis in patients with acute myocardial infarction. *Br Med J* **324:** 1328–31

Quinn C (2003) Infusion devices: understanding the patient perspective to avoid errors. *Prof Nurse* **19:** 79–83

Randolph AG, Cook DJ, Gonzales CA, Andrew M (1998) Benefit of heparin in peripheral venous and arterial catheters: systematic review and meta-analysis of randomised controlled trials. *Br Med J* **316:** 969–75

Raybould LM (2001) Disposable non-sterile gloves: a policy for appropriate usage. *Br J Nurs* **10:** 1135–41

Rourke C, Bates C, Read RC (2001) Poor hospital infection control practice in venepuncture and use of tourniquets. *J Hosp Infect* **49**(1): 59–61

Scales K (1997) Practical and professional aspects of IV therapy. *Prof Nurse* **12**(Suppl 8): 53–5

Serious Hazards of Transfusion (2003) *Summary of Annual Report 2003*. SHOT, Manchester

Useful website

ECG Web-Based Computer Assisted Learning
www.hls.dmu.ac.uk/teaching/manwar/

Chapter 6

Gastrointestinal system

Abdominal paracentesis

Abdominal paracentesis is used to drain an abnormal collection of fluid from the abdomen. A catheter is placed through the abdominal muscles into the peritoneal cavity.

Reasons for the procedure

⌘ Collection of ascitic fluid for analysis by microbiology, histology and cytology
⌘ Drainage of fluid to relieve physical pressure within the abdomen and on the diaphragm created by a large collection of ascitic fluid. This also improves the patient's physical appearance
⌘ Administration of drugs or agents into the peritoneal cavity. This may be chemotherapy or anti-bacterial agents (Evans et al, 2003).

Pre-procedure

Equipment required

Some units provide a specific abdominal paracentesis pack. If not, the following equipment is required:

⌘ Incontinence sheet to protect bed linen
⌘ Dressing trolley, sterile dressing pack, sterile towels and drapes to create a sterile field
⌘ Cleansing agent such as chlorhexidine or iodine to clean the patient's skin
⌘ Sterile gloves for aseptic technique
⌘ Local anaesthetic such as lignocaine to numb the skin, subcutaneous tissue and muscle
⌘ A variety of sizes of needles to inject local anaesthetic, starting with the smallest size and continuing through to larger sizes so all layers of the abdominal wall are effectively anaesthetized
⌘ 5 ml syringes
⌘ Scalpel to cut through skin

⌘ Peritoneal trocar catheter or other suitable cannula to allow for drainage of fluid from the abdominal cavity

⌘ Sterile receiver to collect ascitic drainage initially

⌘ Specimen pots to send samples of fluid to laboratories

⌘ Sutures to secure trocar catheter *in situ* if required

⌘ Three-way tap and connector to facilitate drainage

⌘ 50 ml bladder syringe to connect to three-way tap and connector to facilitate drainage

⌘ Large, sterile drainage bag may be used as an alternative to three-way connector to collect drainage, especially if trocar catheter remains *in situ*

⌘ Clamps to clamp or restrict flow/drainage of ascitic fluid, especially if trocar catheter remaining *in situ* beyond 24–48 hours

⌘ Suitable dressing to protect site

⌘ Non-sterile jug to measure amount of drainage post-procedure

⌘ Waste-disposal sack — biohazard

⌘ Sharps bins.

Specific patient preparation required

⌘ Clinical observations of temperature, pulse, respirations, blood pressure, weight and girth to act as a baseline to assess changes in the patient's condition

⌘ Ask the patient to empty his/her bladder to ensure that there is a reduced risk of accidental perforation of the bladder when the trocar catheter is inserted

⌘ Ensure the patient is comfortable lying as prone as possible in the bed

⌘ Protect the bed linen with incontinence sheets placed under and at the side of the patient

⌘ The patient's abdomen is exposed and the abdomen is palpated to select the most suitable site for abdominal paracentesis.

During the procedure

⌘ The nurse assists the doctor to unpack all the required sterile equipment. The doctor washes his/her hands and dons sterile gloves

⌘ The patient's abdomen is cleaned with the cleansing solution

⌘ A sterile field is created on the patient's abdomen by placement of the sterile sheets and drapes

⌘ Local anaesthetic is injected into the skin, starting with the smallest size needle for subcutaneous tissue and continuing with larger needles for the muscular layer of the abdominal wall

⌘ Once the local anaesthetic has taken effect, a small incision is made into the abdomen with a scalpel. The trocar catheter is inserted via this incision

⌘ Ascitic fluid may be drained directly from the trocar catheter with fluid collected into the receiver. Alternatively, the trocar catheter may be connected to a closed continuous drainage system. If the trocar catheter is to remain *in situ*, it is secured in place with sutures. The site is dressed with a sterile suitable dressing.

Post–procedure

⌘ The equipment used during the procedure is disposed of as per local policy
⌘ Observations of pulse, respirations and blood pressure are taken and recorded. Observations are repeated as clinically indicated
⌘ If the trocar catheter remains *in situ*, the patient requires information about how to safely mobilize without dislodging the catheter
⌘ The quantity, colour and consistency of the ascitic fluid that is drained should be noted. A strict fluid balance chart should be maintained to record loss from the abdominal paracentesis and via the closed drainage system. This is to try to prevent hypovolaemic shock and abdominal pain by unobstructed drainage. Up to 5 litres of drainage is acceptable, providing the patient does not have any adverse reactions to fluid loss
⌘ Measurements of weight and girth assist the healthcare team to assess fluid loss and fluid balance overall. The healthcare team will need to ensure that the patient does not become dehydrated or have an imbalance of electrolytes caused by removal of fluid from the abdominal cavity. Intravenous fluids and electrolyte replacement may need to be considered. The patient requires information about the findings from the test and how this will be reflected in the care plan
⌘ Monitor for complications (*Box 6.1*).

Box 6.1: Complications of abdominal paracentesis

Pain at insertion site

Generalized abdominal pain caused by shift of a large quantity of fluid

Infection of the insertion site

Leakage of fluid around the insertion site

Displacement of the trocar catheter and drainage system

Haemorrhage

Perforation of the bladder or other abdominal organs

Shock/dehydration and electrolyte imbalance caused by fluid loss

---

Compression balloon tamponade

Compression balloon tamponade involves the insertion of a multiple-port tube into the stomach via the mouth. Compression tamponade can involve attaching the tube to weights designed to use traction techniques to pull the inflated gastric balloon up against the cardia of the stomach.

This increases the compression pressure on bleeding varices. The use of a compression balloon tube assists the interprofessional healthcare team to manage the patient's symptom of bleeding varices. It is not a cure or long-term treatment for varices, but may gain valuable time to stabilize the patient to allow for later endoscopic techniques.

Reasons for the procedure

- Aspiration of blood via the gastric and oesophageal ports
- Delivery of medications via the gastric port
- Compression of oesophageal varices.

Pre-procedure

Equipment required

- Lubrication jelly
- Protective/waterproof pads for the trolley/bed/bed linen
- Clamps to allow ports/balloons to be clamped safely
- Magill forceps to pass the tube down the back of the throat
- Spigots to cap off ports
- Gauze to grip the lubricated tube securely
- Compression balloon tube, preferably cooled in the fridge until use to ensure it is slightly rigid and easier to pass
- Bladder syringes to aspirate blood from the oesophageal/gastric ports and insert air into the oesophageal/gastric balloons
- Plastic jugs for collection of aspirated blood
- Manometer to measure balloon pressures
- Non-sterile gloves and plastic aprons to adhere to universal precautions
- Traction equipment: weight, cord, strong adhesive tape, traction beams if used
- Observation charts
- Fluid balance charts.

Specific patient preparation required

- Consider whether the patient requires sedation to assist with passing of the tube (usually a small dose of a benzodiazepine)
- Ensure adequate supplies of intravenous synthetic plasma expanders in case of excessive haemorrhage/hypovolaemic shock
- Baseline observations of temperature, blood pressure, pulse, respirations, peripheral oxygen saturations, central venous pressure, neurological observations and capillary blood sugar level.

These observations act as baseline from which improvement or deterioration of the patient's condition can be assessed
⌘ Assemble all the equipment needed, checking the compression balloon tube to ensure that inflation balloons and aspiration ports are all in good working order.

During the procedure

⌘ Lay the patient on his/her left side, to allow for easier placement of the tube into the stomach via the oesophagus
⌘ The tube should be lubricated and passed via the oesophagus into the stomach. The tube can be passed nasogastrically or orogastrically. The orogastric route is the commonest route
⌘ The tube will be advanced to its full length
⌘ Once the tube is in place, the gastric balloon is inflated with 300 ml air. The tube is gently pulled back until resistance is felt. This indicates that the balloon is in place at the oesophageal–gastric junction
⌘ The balloon requires spigotting off. A clamp is also used to ensure that the balloon cannot deflate accidentally. If the patient becomes distressed or complains of chest pain, inflation of the gastric balloon may have occurred within the oesophagus. The gastric balloon requires deflation, repositioning, re-inflating and position rechecking
⌘ The compression balloon tube's position is confirmed via X-ray. If the tube is correctly positioned, the oesophageal balloon may be inflated with air, spigotted off and clamped. Pressure within the oesophageal balloon is measured with a manometer and is usually up to 40 mmHg. The oesophageal balloon requires deflation for 5 minutes every hour to prevent tissue necrosis (Smith, 2004). During this time the traction weight is also removed
⌘ Entries within the patient's notes are made to indicate tube batch number, insertion length and inflation pressures/amounts of air for the gastric and oesophageal balloons
⌘ The gastric and oesophageal ports are aspirated to remove any blood that has haemorrhaged from the varices. Any fluid loss is recorded on the fluid balance chart.

Post-procedure

⌘ Observe for complications (*Box 6.2*)

Box 6.2: Complications of compression balloon tamponade
Rupture of the oesophagus
Aspiration of blood into the lungs
Tissue necrosis from pressure from the oesophageal balloon
Airway obstruction should the compression balloon tube position slip

⌘ Emergencies — should the patient become distressed or have difficulties in breathing or require resuscitation, the compression tamponade balloon can be removed easily and rapidly. The gastric and oesophageal balloons can be deflated rapidly by cutting through the tube. The tube can then removed

⌘ Communication — the patient will be able to speak but communication will be impaired. The patient requires empathy to assist him/her to express his/her needs or fears

⌘ Ensure the call bell is to hand

⌘ Observation/monitoring — observations are likely to be required every 15–30 minutes until the patient's condition stabilizes. Observations can then be recorded each hour until the tube is removed

⌘ Oral hygiene — the patient is unable to eat or drink while the tube is *in situ*. A nil-by-mouth sign should be displayed. The patient requires oral assessment, assistance with oral care, plus lubrication of the lips to prevent drying/cracking. This is particularly important as the patient is likely to have vomited blood (haematemesis) and may have halitosis

⌘ Administration of medications — most medications may be administered intravenously. Lactulose is likely to be used to ensure that any residual/decaying blood, post-bleeding varices is eliminated. Lactulose may be administered via the gastric port of the compression balloon, providing it is carefully and thoroughly flushed through to prevent any potential blockage. Alternatively, lactulose may be administered rectally in the form of an enema

⌘ Preparation for further tests and investigations — the patient is likely to return to the endoscopy unit after 12–48 hours. This will be to remove the tube and endoscopically view the varices. Other mechanical methods of treating the varices may then commence.

Endoscopic procedures

An endoscopic procedure involves the insertion of a fibreoptic scope, which consists of a firm, but flexible, plastic tube with a controllable end bearing a light. The tube has additional channels for introducing air and for therapeutic procedures. There are a variety of endoscopic techniques, including:

⌘ *Gastroscopy* — examination of the upper gastrointestinal (GI) tract including the oesophagus, stomach and first part of the duodenum

⌘ *Flexible sigmoidoscopy* — examination of the rectum and sigmoid colon

⌘ *Colonoscopy* — examination of the rectum, colon and terminal ileum.

Reasons for the procedure

Gastroscopy

⌘ To diagnose upper GI tract disorders such as hiatus hernias, oesophagitis, gastritis, gastric ulceration, duodenal ulceration, oesophageal carcinoma and gastric carcinoma

⌘ Therapeutic techniques such as dilatation of strictures in the oesophagus or at the oesophageal–gastric junction, banding/sclerosing of oesophageal varices

⌘ Supportive techniques such as placement of feeding tubes.

Flexible sigmoidoscopy

⌘ To diagnose lower GI tract disorders such as rectal bleeding, altered bowel habit
⌘ To assess for disease such as inflammatory bowel disease and colorectal cancer
⌘ To undertake therapeutic techniques such as removal of polyps with snaring techniques and electrocautery.

Colonoscopy

⌘ To examine the entire length of the colon and terminal ileum
⌘ To diagnose lower GI tract disorders such as rectal bleeding, altered bowel habit
⌘ To assess for disease such as inflammatory bowel disease and colorectal cancer
⌘ To undertake therapeutic techniques such as removal of polyps with snaring techniques and electrocautery.

Pre-procedure

Equipment required

⌘ Water-based lubricant
⌘ Medications for sedation as prescribed
⌘ Oxygen and mask
⌘ Suction unit
⌘ Gloves
⌘ Apron
⌘ Goggles
⌘ Mouth guard
⌘ Incontinence pads as necessary
⌘ Pre-labelled specimen bottles/solution
⌘ Lignocaine spray as required
⌘ Patient-monitoring equipment for blood pressure, pulse and oxygen saturation
⌘ Appropriate scope for procedure following manufacturer's guidelines
⌘ Related attachments (suction, water port, light source, biopsy, diathermy) following manufacturer's guidelines
⌘ Audiovisual recording equipment following manufacturer's guidelines.

Specific patient preparation required

Preparation of the GI tract. The GI tract needs to be clear of fluids and solids if endoscopic techniques are to be employed safely and effectively. Preparation of the GI tract takes the following form:

⌘ *Gastroscopy* — the patient needs to be made nil-by-mouth 6 hours before the test to ensure that the stomach is empty

⌘ *Flexible sigmoidoscopy* — the patient requires a phosphate enema before the test to ensure that the rectum and sigmoid colon are free from faeces

⌘ *Colonoscopy* — the patient requires a mixed regimen of light diet/free fluids and bowel-preparation solutions. The patient requires clear instructions on how to use the bowel preparation solution correctly. This ensures that the entire colon is free of faeces.

Observations

Observations of temperature, pulse, respirations, blood pressure, peripheral oxygen saturations and weight are recorded to act as a baseline from which the patient's condition can be assessed. This is prior to commencing endoscopic techniques and to measure for any potential problems or deterioration during and after the tests. Weight is required to assess the correct level of sedation or analgesia if required.

During the procedure

Gastroscopy

⌘ The patient has his/her throat sprayed with local anaesthetic such as lignocaine to numb the back of the throat, enabling easier passage of the scope

⌘ Sedation may be given if required. This is usually a benzodiazepine given in incremental doses until the patient is settled but not heavily sedated

⌘ The patient is positioned in the left lateral position to allow for easier inspection of the stomach once the scope is passed

⌘ A mouth guard is employed to ensure that the patient does not bite the scope accidentally and to facilitate removal of oral secretions via suction

⌘ The endoscope is lubricated using a water-soluble lubricant and passed via the oropharynx into the oesophagus and on to the stomach. Biopsies may be taken or therapeutic techniques may be employed. Water is used to flush the end of the endoscope to keep it clear of secretions. Air may be inserted into the patient via the endoscope to assist with viewing of the GI tract

⌘ At the end of gastroscopy, the endoscope is removed slowly and gently.

Flexible sigmoidoscopy

⌘ Sedation may sometimes be required. This is usually a benzodiazepine given in incremental doses until the patient is settled but not heavily sedated

⌘ The patient is positioned in the left lateral position to allow for easier inspection of the rectum and sigmoid colon once the scope is passed

⌘ A digital examination is carried out to check for any obvious obstructions or problems

⌘ The scope is lubricated with a water-soluble lubricant and passed into the rectum. The scope is advanced further into the descending colon, using twists, torsion and advancing/withdrawing to pass smoothly. Biopsies may be taken and therapeutic techniques employed. Water is used to flush the end of the endoscope to keep it clear of secretions. Air may be inserted into the patient via the endoscope to assist with viewing the GI tract

⌘ At the end of flexible sigmoidoscopy, the scope is removed slowly and gently.

Colonoscopy

⌘ Sedation is usually required. Analgesia may also be required. This is usually a benzodiazepine and an opiate such as pethidine. It is given in incremental doses until the patient is settled/pain-free but not heavily sedated

⌘ The patient is positioned in the left lateral position to allow for easier inspection of the rectum and sigmoid colon once the scope is passed

⌘ A digital examination is carried out to check for any obvious obstructions or problems

⌘ The colonoscope is lubricated with a water-soluble lubricant and passed into the rectum. The colonoscope is advanced further into the descending, transverse and ascending colon, using twists, torsion and advancing/withdrawing to pass smoothly. Nursing staff may be required to apply abdominal pressure to assist with insertion of the colonoscope. Biopsies may be taken and therapeutic techniques employed. Water is used to flush the end of the endoscope to keep it clear of secretions. Air may be inserted into the patient via the endoscope to assist with viewing the GI tract

⌘ At the end of colonoscopy, the colonoscope is removed slowly and gently.

Post-procedure

⌘ Observations of pulse, respirations, blood pressure and peripheral oxygen saturations are taken and recorded. These are repeated as clinically indicated, which may be every 15 minutes until the patient's condition is stable

⌘ The patient may be given a drink and small snack once recovered. This will vary according to local policy

⌘ Then the patient can be transferred back to the ward or discharged home into the care of a suitable adult

⌘ Written information on potential post-procedure problems/instructions on when to resume a normal diet/fluids should be provided

⌘ Once recovered from the procedure and fully alert/orientated, the patient requires information about the findings from the test

⌘ Where biopsies or samples have been taken, the patient will need to be reviewed by the healthcare team once the results are available from the laboratory. The nurse should arrange appropriate follow-up for the patient

⌘ Monitor for complications, which may include oversedation/respiratory depression, cardiorespiratory events/emergencies, haemorrhage and perforation.

Gastric lavage

Gastric lavage is the aspiration of stomach contents and washing out of the stomach using a large-bore gastric tube (Smeltzer and Bare, 2000). It is referred to as a stomach washout or stomach pump. It is most frequently used after an overdose of prescribed/non-prescribed drugs and alcohol or other substances. However, its use for the management of overdose remains controversial as gastric lavage is most effective within 1–2 hours of ingestion of substances. Many patients may not present early enough for gastric lavage to be beneficial (Lynch and Robertson, 2003). The procedure may be carried out by suitably trained nurses (Nursing and Midwifery Council, 2002).

Careful management of the patient's airway is required because of the risk of aspiration of stomach contents. Where the patient's airway is compromised, such as in intentional overdose, anaesthetic opinion should be sought as the patient may require endotracheal intubation. Local policy should be followed.

Reasons for the procedure

⌘ To empty the stomach of ingested substances to prevent absorption
⌘ As part of the management for intentional overdose where the substance ingested is not absorbed by activated charcoal (Littlejohn, 2004)
⌘ To empty the stomach for gastroscopy
⌘ Key contraindications for gastric lavage include ingestion of petroleum distillates and corrosive substances.

Pre-procedure

Equipment required

⌘ Emergency oxygen, suction and cardiac arrest trolley to hand in case of potential emergency
⌘ Incontinence sheet to protect bed linen
⌘ Non-sterile gloves and plastic aprons to protect from the potential risk of accidental spillage of gastric contents on the nurse's uniform
⌘ Water-based lubrication jelly to lubricate gastric tube for insertion
⌘ Lignocaine throat spray — local anaesthetic for the oropharynx
⌘ Mouth guard to prevent the patient biting on the gastric tube
⌘ Gastric tube — a large-bore gastric tube
⌘ Funnel and connector to allow delivery of fluid
⌘ Jugs to contain tap water
⌘ Tap water at a tepid temperature to prevent shock/discomfort of cold water being inserted into the stomach
⌘ Bucket or large receiver to collect stomach contents/fluids after drainage from the stomach

⌘ Specimen pots — large size
⌘ Wipes, soap, towel to clean the patient post-procedure
⌘ Waste-disposal sack — biohazard
⌘ Activated charcoal may be used to absorb any residual substances
⌘ Oral hygiene equipment to freshen the oral mucosa.

Specific patient preparation required

⌘ Clinical observations of temperature, pulse, respirations, blood pressure and peripheral saturations are recorded
⌘ Consideration of capillary blood glucose levels and use of the Glasgow Coma Scale/neurological observations should be reviewed, especially if the patient has fluctuating levels of consciousness
⌘ The patient's clothes must be loose on the top half of his/her body
⌘ Ensure the patient is comfortable lying in the left lateral position with knees drawn up towards the chest. This pools contents in the stomach and prevents the continuing passage of stomach contents into the duodenum
⌘ Assess the length of gastric tube to be used, measuring from the bridge of the nose to the xiphoid process
⌘ Local anaesthetic throat spray is used if appropriate
⌘ Protect the bed linen with incontinence sheets placed under the patient's shoulder, neck and face.

During the procedure

⌘ The gastric tube and funnel are connected together
⌘ The gastric tube is lubricated and is passed into the stomach via the mouth, oropharynx and oesophagus
⌘ A mouth guard may be used to prevent the tube from being accidentally bitten
⌘ The patient is asked to try and assist placement of the tube by swallowing the gastric tube as it is advanced. The patient may find the procedure unpleasant
⌘ The nurse should observe for any difficulties in breathing, cyanosis or stridor, indicating that the tube has passed into the trachea rather than the oesophagus
⌘ Confirmation of correct placement positioning of the tube may be required by X-ray. The placement of the gastric tube is also confirmed by aspiration of gastric contents. The entire stomach contents are aspirated. The initial specimens of gastric contents are collected in specimen pots and retained for pathological testing
⌘ The head of the bed or trolley is lowered as this will assist gravity and the siphoning effect during the lavage
⌘ Tepid tap water is inserted into the stomach via the funnel/gastric tube, usually about 200 ml at a time. Gravity is used to feed the water into the stomach, with the funnel held above the patient's head. Before the funnel has completely drained of water, the funnel is dropped down and inverted over the receiver or bucket. This is repeated until the fluid obtained from the stomach runs clear

⌘ Activated charcoal (a powder mixed with water to form a slurry that can be administered via a 50 ml bladder syringe into the gastric tube) may be administered via the gastric tube to prevent further absorption of substances.

Post-procedure

⌘ If an endotracheal tube has been inserted for the procedure, this may be removed once the medical/anaesthetic staff are satisfied that the patient can maintain a patent airway
⌘ Assist the patient to maintain his/her oral hygiene needs and to dress post-procedure
⌘ Have the call bell to hand so that the patient may summon assistance if required
⌘ Make a note of the amount of fluid used for the gastric lavage and compare this to the amount of stomach contents/fluid drained. Also note the quantity, consistency and colour of stomach contents and any obvious tablets or substances in the patient's notes
⌘ Record clinical observations to assess for any change in the patient's condition.

Complications

Complications for gastric lavage include:

⌘ Aspiration of stomach contents
⌘ Abdominal pain/cramping secondary to gastric lavage
⌘ Perforation of the oesophagus/stomach
⌘ Water intoxication caused by absorption of the water from the stomach.

Liver biopsy

Liver biopsy is a procedure to gain a sample of liver tissue for examination in the laboratory to assist with diagnosis or assessment of liver disease (Evans et al, 2003). Liver biopsy may be undertaken on the ward, but many centres use the facilities of the X-ray/radiology department to use ultrasound or image-intensification screening techniques to assist with safe placement of the biopsy needle.

Reasons for the procedure

⌘ To obtain a biopsy for investigation.

Pre-procedure

Equipment required

- ⌘ Incontinence sheet to protect bed linen
- ⌘ Dressing trolley, dressing pack, sterile towels/drapes to create a sterile field
- ⌘ Cleansing agent such as chlorhexidine or iodine to clean the patient's skin
- ⌘ Sterile gloves for aseptic technique
- ⌘ Local anaesthetic such as lignocaine to numb the skin, subcutaneous tissue/muscle
- ⌘ A variety of sizes of needles to inject local anaesthetic, starting with the smallest size and continuing through to larger sizes until all layers of the abdominal wall are effectively anaesthetized
- ⌘ Fine-bore needle biopsy for fine-needle aspiration (FNA) to obtain a sample of liver tissue, or large-bore biopsy needle or biopsy gun (Trucut or Bard Biopsy Gun) for large-bore needle aspiration (LNA) to gain liver tissue sample
- ⌘ Specimen pots to send samples of fluid to the laboratories
- ⌘ Sutures to close puncture site
- ⌘ Suitable dressing to protect site
- ⌘ Waste-disposal sack — biohazard
- ⌘ Sharps bins.

Specific patient preparation required

- ⌘ Clinical observations of temperature, pulse, respirations, blood pressure and peripheral saturations are recorded to act as a baseline to assess changes in the patient's condition
- ⌘ Some centres require the patient to be nil-by-mouth for 4 hours before the procedure. This is to try to reduce any nausea and potential for vomiting during the procedure
- ⌘ The patient requires blood samples of group/cross-matching samples (in case of haemorrhage during or after the procedure) and clotting studies to be taken. The results of these must be checked before the liver biopsy
- ⌘ If the clotting studies are abnormal, intravenous vitamin K 10 mg may be administered to reduce the patient's clotting time. Blood samples for clotting studies should then be rechecked
- ⌘ The doctor should explain the procedure to the patient and practise the breathing techniques required during the procedure
- ⌘ A small dose of sedation such as a bendodiazepine may be used. However, the doctor will require the patient's cooperation during the test so the patient should not be heavily sedated
- ⌘ Ensure the patient is comfortable lying prone in the bed with his/her abdomen exposed.

During the procedure

- ⌘ The nurse assists the doctor to unpack all the required sterile equipment
- ⌘ The doctor washes his/her hands and dons sterile gloves

⌘ The patient places his/her right hand under his/her head so that the right arm is free of the abdominal area

⌘ The patient's abdomen (right upper epigastric quadrant) is cleaned with the cleansing solution. A sterile field is created on the patient's abdomen by placement of the sterile sheets and drapes

⌘ Local anaesthetic is injected into the skin starting with the smallest size needle for subcutaneous tissue and continuing with larger size needles for the muscular layer of the abdominal wall. The local anaesthetic requires time to take effect

⌘ The doctor asks the patient to coordinate his/her breathing with the insertion of the biopsy needle. The patient is required to inspire and hold a large amount of air as the doctor inserts the biopsy needle. The inspired held breath assists the liver to lie close to the wall of the abdomen

⌘ For FNA — the biopsy needle is inserted directly though the skin and a sample of liver tissue is taken

⌘ For LNA — a small incision is made into the abdomen with a scalpel. The biopsy needle is inserted via this incision. A larger sample of liver tissue is collected

⌘ The biopsy needle is withdrawn and pressure is applied to the insertion site; continuous application of pressure may be required for up to 20 minutes to ensure effective clotting has occurred at the biopsy site

⌘ For LNA the incision is closed with a suture

⌘ The site is dressed with a suitable sterile dressing.

Post-procedure

⌘ Dispose of equipment according to local policy

⌘ Clinical observations of pulse, respirations, blood pressure and peripheral oxygen saturations are taken and recorded. Initially observations are repeated every 15 minutes for 2 hours, then reduced to half-hourly for 2 hours, then reduced to hourly for 4 hours and then recorded as clinically indicated

⌘ The nurse should also check the incision site and its dressing with the recording of the observations. This is to assess for any potential haemorrhage from the liver biopsy site

⌘ The patient may drink when he/she feels comfortable. Assistance with change of position in bed, elimination and other activities may be required during the initial 4 hours post-procedure/during bed rest. The patient may eat/mobilize after 4 hours

⌘ The patient requires information about the findings from the test and how this will be reflected within his/her plan of care. The nurse needs to make arrangements for removal of the suture in 7–10 days

⌘ Monitor for potential complications (*Box 6.3*).

Box 6.3: Complications of liver biopsy

Pain at the insertion site

Generalized abdominal pain caused by biopsy of the liver

Infection of the insertion site

Leakage of fluid/blood around the insertion site

Haemorrhage

Damage to the liver or other abdominal organs if the biopsy needle is not carefully inserted

---

Managing stomas

'Stoma' is the Greek word for mouth or opening, and is a passageway that has been constructed by a surgeon through the abdominal wall using a section of bowel as an exit for faeces or urine when the urinary or colonic tract beyond the position of the stoma is no longer viable.

A stoma can be formed in any part of the gastrointestinal tract, at any age, for a variety of reasons, including those listed in *Box 6.4*.

Box 6.4: Reasons for formation of a stoma

Congenital anomalies

Inflammatory bowel disease

Familial polyposis coli

Bowel cancer

Bladder cancer

Other pelvic cancers, e.g. gynaecological

Diverticular disease

Trauma, e.g. after a road traffic accident

Neurological conditions such as spina bifida

Radiation damage

Colovaginal/colovesical fistula

There are three basic types of eliminating stomas:

⌘ *Colostomy* — an opening into the large colon (large bowel)
⌘ *Ileostomy* — an opening into the ileum (small intestine)
⌘ *Urostomy* — an opening into the urinary tract.

Reasons for the procedure

⌘ To ensure that the correct appliance for the patient's needs has been fitted
⌘ To monitor the condition and function of the stoma
⌘ To secure a leak-proof, comfortable-fitting appliance
⌘ To provide opportunities for discussion and to explore patient concerns
⌘ To identify and resolve potential problems
⌘ To assist patients with the physical and psychological adaptation of life with a stoma
⌘ To teach patients about the care of their stoma and the surrounding skin.

Pre-procedure: emptying an existing appliance

Equipment required

⌘ Gloves
⌘ Plastic apron
⌘ Soft wipes
⌘ Paper hand towels
⌘ Basin or receptacle for warm water (hand hot)
⌘ Disposal bag
⌘ Measuring jug.

Specific patient preparation required

⌘ Forewarn patient of the potential for malodour
⌘ Establish level of patient involvement.

During the procedure

⌘ Wash hands, wear gloves and apron
⌘ Place a clean hand towel beneath the patient's appliance to protect against any drips if the effluent is fluid

⌘ Place the jug beneath the end of the appliance, release integral clip or remove clip, drain the contents of the appliance into the jug

⌘ Clean the bottom of the appliance using wipes and warm water. Re-attach clip to the appliance. If an integral clip is used, clean with warm water and close following the manufacturer's instructions

⌘ Measure output, note colour, consistency and volume; mentally note the presence of flatus in the pouch

⌘ Cover jug, remove effluent and dispose in the sluice following local procedure

⌘ Dispose of soiled wipes as per hospital policy

⌘ The frequency that an appliance requires emptying will be dependent on the output.

Post-procedure

⌘ Record in fluid chart

⌘ Abnormalities such as high output — inform senior nursing or medical staff if necessary.

Pre-procedure: changing of appliance

Equipment required

⌘ Wipes

⌘ Paper hand towels

⌘ Basin or receptacle for warm water. The temperature of the water should be hand hot

⌘ New appliance with integral clip or, if necessary, separate clip

⌘ Disposal bag

⌘ Measuring jug

⌘ Template (cut to size — using sharp scissors cut out the shape of the stoma, taking care not to puncture the appliance. If possible, use curved scissors. Smooth out any rough edges by running your finger around the aperture of the flange)

⌘ Scissors

⌘ Disposable gloves

⌘ Plastic apron.

Specific patient preparation required

⌘ Warn patient when removing the appliance as there may be some pulling of the skin

⌘ Forewarn of potential spillage.

During the procedure

⌘ Always empty bag before changing it if applicable

⌘ To remove the bag start at the top of the appliance (there is normally a tab at the top of the bag to indicate the starting point). Gently ease the bag away from the skin by using the finger and thumb of one hand while exerting gentle pressure on the skin with the other hand. Work towards the bottom of the flange and avoid tugging or pulling of the appliance

⌘ Place soiled appliance in disposal bag (clinical waste bag)

⌘ Wipe the stoma with a wet tissue, removing excess faeces or mucus

⌘ Wash and dry the surrounding parastomal skin with warm water

⌘ Observe the stoma's colour; observe for parastomal skin soreness, ulceration or any other abnormalities. Check mucocutaneous junction (where the stoma is sutured to the skin) for signs of dehiscence and infection

⌘ Measure the stoma using the template

⌘ Ensure that the parastomal skin is thoroughly dry; apply clean appliance according to manufacturer's instructions, ensuring that the inner edge of the appliance makes contact with the skin

⌘ Secure bag as appropriate

⌘ Dispose of the soiled appliances, wipes and bag, in line with hospital policy

⌘ Wash hands.

Post-procedure

⌘ Offer the patient handwashing facilities

⌘ Ensure that the appliance feels comfortable

⌘ Replace patient's appliance equipment

⌘ Record output in fluid chart

⌘ Any abnormalities — inform senior nursing or medical staff if necessary.

Distal loop washout

Distal loop bowel washouts are carried out to 'wash out' the distal or lower part of the bowel that has been defunctioned by either a loop or divided colostomy (*Figure 6.1*).

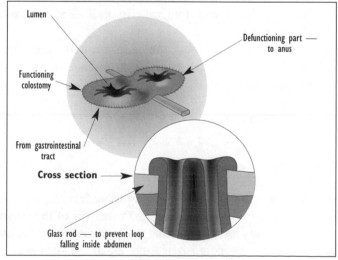

Figure 6.1: Loop colostomy

Fluid is run into the distal opening of the colostomy using an irrigation set and cone. The fluid passes along the colon and is passed per rectum (MacPhail, 2003). This is a safe procedure; however, it is contraindicated in cases where there is a known obstructing lesion. Distal loop washout should only be carried out when prescribed by a doctor. Before the washout, the defunctioned distal loop should be identified by inserting a gloved finger into the outlet of the stoma.

Identification of the distal loop

This is anatomically to the left of the stoma but may be twisted; digital examination of both openings should reveal faeces in the proximal colon and mucus in the distal loop (MacPhail, 2003). Alternatively, the patient may be able to identify the functioning outlet.

Reasons for the procedure

⌘ To clean and prepare the bowel for surgery preoperatively, for example reversal of stoma
⌘ Symptom relief, e.g. in cases where there is overproduction of mucus caused by tumour in the rectum or inadequate bowel surgery preoperatively
⌘ To clear the lower bowel before radiological investigation.

Equipment required

⌘ Disposable gloves
⌘ Plastic apron
⌘ Lubricant gel
⌘ Soft wipes
⌘ Paper hand towels
⌘ Basin or receptacle for warm water
⌘ New appliance with integral clip or, if necessary, separate clip
⌘ Disposal bag
⌘ Irrigation set (reservoir, tubing, cone, irrigation, sleeve)
⌘ Warm water — approximately 1 litre hand-hot water
⌘ Incontinence pad
⌘ Commode
⌘ Drip stand or hook.

Preparation of equipment

⌘ Prepare irrigation set following manufacturer's instructions
⌘ Measure 1 litre of fluid into the reservoir of the irrigation set and run water through the tubing to remove any air bubbles that may be present. Close the clamp until ready to commence procedure
⌘ Attach the prepared irrigation set to the drip stand/hook. This should be at patient's shoulder height.

Specific patient preparation required

⌘ Forewarn patient of potential discomfort as fluid is being introduced, as well as leakage of fluid per rectum for some time
⌘ Drain and remove the soiled appliance
⌘ Clean and wash stoma/parastomal skin
⌘ Fit the irrigation sleeve over the stoma, secure belt, leaving the top of the sleeve open
⌘ Close the end of the irrigation sleeve using integral clip.

During the procedure

⌘ Patient should be sat on a commode/toilet/bedpan
⌘ Insert a gloved finger into the defunctioned outlet to relax and to assess direction of the bowel
⌘ Lubricate the stoma and the end of the cone. Gently insert cone into the stoma
⌘ Release the clip and run the water through at a steady rate. A litre of fluid should take approximately 5–10 minutes to run through. Initially this should be slowly to ensure patency of the bowel and that fluid has been passed rectally. The rate can then be adjusted (MacPhail, 2003). Continue until the fluid runs clear
⌘ If the water will not run freely the cone may be blocked with faeces or resting against the mucosa
⌘ If the water flow is too slow the bowel may have gone into spasm
⌘ If the patient experiences abdominal pain, it may be as a result of the water running in too quickly or cold — adjust rate and temperature as necessary
⌘ Remove cone from the stoma
⌘ Close the top of the sleeve
⌘ If there is no further drainage per rectum after 10 minutes, remove irrigation sleeve
⌘ Clean and dry the parastomal skin
⌘ Apply new appliance, ensuring that this feels comfortable
⌘ Offer the patient washing facilities and assist the patient, if required.

Post-procedure

⌘ Sit the patient on an incontinence pad
⌘ Dispose of soiled equipment, wipes, appliance as per hospital policy
⌘ Clean irrigation equipment — this can be reused for the same patient
⌘ Replace patient's appliance equipment
⌘ Record output in fluid chart
⌘ Record result of washout in nursing documentation
⌘ Monitor for complications — distal loop washout of the bowel may cause a drop in blood pressure and pulse, causing the patient to feel faint (MacPhail, 2003).

Giving an enema via a stoma

The administration of enemas can also prove to be problematic because of the lack of sphincter muscles, and any fluid that is introduced into the stoma will be expelled quickly.

When administrating enemas it is advisable to use a two-piece appliance, fitting the baseplate before insertion of the enema. Once the enema has been administered, the bag can be clipped to the base plate.

Enemas should only be given if prescribed by a doctor or nurse prescriber.

Reasons for the procedure

- ⌘ To empty the bowel of faeces.

Equipment required

- ⌘ Stoma bag
- ⌘ Enema as prescribed
- ⌘ Water-based lubricant
- ⌘ Disposal bag
- ⌘ Gloves.

Specific patient preparation required

- ⌘ Forewarn the patient of potential discomfort and increased bowel activity.

During the procedure

- ⌘ Drain and remove the soiled appliance
- ⌘ Fit new appliance (two-piece) baseplate only (drainable bag is fitted after administration of the enema)
- ⌘ Lubricate the stoma
- ⌘ Insert a lubricated gloved finger into outlet to relax and to assess direction of the bowel
- ⌘ Ensure the enema is warmed to body temperature
- ⌘ Insert the nozzle into the stoma and squeeze the fluid gently and slowly
- ⌘ Fit bag to baseplate
- ⌘ Dispose of soiled equipment.

Post-procedure

⌘ Monitor and document result
⌘ Advise patient about dietary change
⌘ Review drugs that may have caused the problem
⌘ Change bag as necessary.

Student skill laboratory activity

⌘ Assemble equipment required to change a stoma bag

⌘ Practise applying a bag on a manikin with a stoma

⌘ Cut the template to fit around the stoma.

Nasogastric tubes

A nasogastric tube (NG) is a plastic tube that is inserted through the nose or mouth and travels from the nose/mouth to the stomach. NG tubes are available in many sizes (French gauge or Fg) and for different purposes. The choice of tube is dependent on the patient's clinical condition. For enteral feeding, a fine-bore 5–8 Fg NG tube is the tube of choice. For continuous stomach aspiration or the administration of high-fibre feed and drugs, a larger bore feeding tube is required (12–14 Fg) (Stroud et al, 2003).

Reasons for the procedure

⌘ To instil liquids and foods
⌘ To withdraw gastric contents from the stomach because of bowel obstruction, paralytic ileus.

Pre-procedure

Equipment required

⌘ Nasogastric tube of appropriate size
⌘ Apron
⌘ Clinical waste bag

⌘ Tray
⌘ Sterile water
⌘ Hypoallergenic tape or appropriate securing fixative (some manufacturers include a self-adhesive fixative)
⌘ Glass of water and a straw where appropriate
⌘ Sterile syringe 50 ml — use once only
⌘ Gloves
⌘ pH strips
⌘ Spigot
⌘ Drainage bag.

Specific patient preparation required

⌘ If possible, arrange a signal by which the patient can communicate if he/she wants to stop, for example by raising his/her hands
⌘ Ensure that the patient is comfortable and sitting as upright as possible, supported with plenty of pillows
⌘ Check the patient has patent nostrils. Ask him/her to blow his/her nose first — this will help to identify obstructions liable to prevent insertion (McConnell, 1997)
⌘ If the patient is unconscious, he/she should be placed in a left fetal position with the head tilted forward. This facilitates the passage of the tube into the oesophagus.

During the procedure

⌘ Mark the tube at a distance equal to that from the xiphisternum to the nose via the earlobe (50–60 cm) (Stroud et al, 2003). Mark with tape and record in the nursing notes
⌘ Check that the guidewire moves freely, without kinks (only for fine-bore NG tube). Lubricate the proximal end of the tube with sterile water
⌘ Insert the rounded end of the NG tube into the clearest nostril and slide it backwards and inwards along the floor of the nose to the nasopharynx. If any resistance is met, withdraw the tube and insert into the other nostril or try the same nostril but use a slightly different angle. As the tube passes down the nasopharynx, ask the patient to mimic swallowing. (If patient is allowed fluid, a sip of water can be given to assist with swallowing.) Advance the tube 5–10 cm as the patient swallows. Do this until the predetermined mark on the tube has been reached
⌘ If the patient is distressed, develops severe ear pain, starts to cough or becomes cyanosed, withdraw the tube immediately (Arslantas et al, 2001)
⌘ Check tube position by using a 50 ml syringe and aspirate 3 ml fluid with gentle suction. If aspiration is difficult, change the patient's position; or if safe to do so, give the patient a drink to dilute the stomach contents. The pH of the stomach contents is usually between 3–4 (Metheny et al, 1994). Bronchial secretions have a pH greater >6
⌘ Place the aspirate onto pH strips. A pH of ≤4 shows that the tip of the tube is in the correct position. If the pH is >4, retry after 1 hour

✼ An X-ray is required if unsure as to whether the tube is in the correct place. The X-ray should be reported by a radiologist or registrar and the position of the tip of the feeding tube documented in the patient notes

✼ Secure NG tube

✼ Attach spigot or drainage bag as requested.

Post-procedure

✼ Dispose of equipment as per local policy

✼ Complete nursing documentation

✼ Aspirate NG tube as requested and document

✼ Empty drainage bag and record accordingly

✼ Make patient aware of potential constraints and to avoid pulling NG tube out

✼ Observe for potential complications (*Box 6.5*)

Box 6.5: Potential complications of NG tube insertion

Monitor for sore mouth, thirst, swallowing difficulties and hoarseness (Duncan and Silk, 2001)

Check for local pressure effects from the tube, such as nasal erosion, abscess formation, sinusitis and otitis media

Observe for short-term oesophageal damage, such as oesophagitis and ulceration from localized abrasion and gastro-oesophageal reflux (Stroud et al, 2003)

✼ If the patient is receiving antacids, pH results may not be indicative of accurate positioning of the tube.

Student skill laboratory activity

✼ Identify the equipment you would require to insert both a Ryle's and a fine-bore nasogastric tube

✼ Practise how to measure the tube from the xiphisternum to the nose on a manikin.

Nutrition in clinical practice: enteral feeding

Enteral feeding is the delivery of nutrients directly into the gastrointestinal tract via a feeding tube. There are various methods for administering enteral nutrition, and these include tube feeding via nasogastric tube, nasoenteric, nasojejunal, oesophagostomy or percutaneous endoscopic gastrostomy (PEG). Enteral nutrition is available in many forms to suit the individual needs of the patient.

Reasons for the procedure

⌘ Enteral feeding is indicated for those who cannot eat enough to meet their nutritional needs orally, but whose gut is functioning normally (Holmes, 2002)

⌘ For those who are unable to eat for a prolonged period of time, such as the unconscious patient

⌘ Maintains the structure and integrity of the gut (ASPEN, 2002), which is associated with fewer postoperative complications.

Pre-procedure

Equipment required

⌘ Prescription chart
⌘ Prescribed feed
⌘ Gloves
⌘ Apron
⌘ Nutritional giving set
⌘ Feeding pump
⌘ pH strips
⌘ 50 ml catheter tip syringe
⌘ Receiver
⌘ Drip stand
⌘ Fluid balance chart
⌘ Prescribed sterile water.

Specific patient preparation required

⌘ Inform the patient that his/her next feed is due and establish if he/she has experienced any problems in relation to the feed (*Box 6.6*).

Box 6.6: Common problems associated with enteral feeding

Diarrhoea

Nausea and vomiting

Fullness

Abdominal pain

Reflux

Coughing or choking

During the procedure

⌘ Assemble necessary equipment and feed
⌘ Disassemble existing nutritional giving set and discard as per local policy (leave feeding tube *in situ*)
⌘ Put on gloves
⌘ Attach the 50 ml catheter tip syringe to the port of the feeding tube
⌘ Confirm position of feeding tube by aspirating an amount of gastrointestinal content and test for pH (ensuring that manufacturer's guidelines are followed)
⌘ Place a small amount of aspirate on the pH strip, note and record if the pH is indicative of the tube being in the correct position. If it is not in the correct position or if you have any doubts, do not proceed — seek medical help
⌘ Aspirate any remaining unabsorbed feed and place into receiver
⌘ Record the volume on a fluid balance chart and note the colour of the aspirate
⌘ The feed should be suspended on the drip stand by the patient's bed
⌘ The pack containing the giving set should be opened. Ensure that the roller clamp is closed. The seals protecting connection points are exposed, and the giving set connected to the bag of feed
⌘ Open the roller clamp on the giving set and prime it. Ensure that the chamber is not more than half full, otherwise the feeding pump is unable to sense the number of drips required to fulfil the prescription
⌘ Once the line has been primed, attach the giving set to the pump as per instructions
⌘ Attach the end of the giving set to the patient's tube or catheter
⌘ Set the volume of feed to be infused and then set the rate of feed to be infused as per prescription. Once satisfied that this is correct, commence the feed
⌘ Specific care for PEG tubes is listed in *Box 6.7*.

Box 6.7: Care of PEG tubes

The tube should be rotated 360° every day to prevent the formation of scar tissue

Check the stoma a minimum of once daily for leakage, redness, signs of breakdown, soreness, excessive movement of the tube

Clean the stoma with soap and water after day 1

Flush the tube before and after every feed in accordance with the prescribed amount.

Post-procedure

⌘ Clear away the clinical waste and dispose of it correctly as per trust policy
⌘ Document the feed on the fluid balance chart. Ensure that the rate of the feed is correct
⌘ Nutritional assessments should be undertaken according to individual need
⌘ Discuss patient management with the nutritional team.

> ### Student skill laboratory activity
>
> ⌘ Identify the different types of feeding tubes, giving set and feeding pumps available
>
> ⌘ Practise assembling the equipment and familiarize yourself with the workings of the feeding pump.

Nutrition in clinical practice: parenteral nutrition

Parenteral nutrition is the intravenous administration of a solution containing the essential nutrients, namely amino acids, glucose, fat, electrolytes, trace elements and vitamins, to meet all daily nutritional requirements of the patient (Hamilton, 2000).

Reasons for the procedure

⌘ If the gastrointestinal tract is unavailable or unable to absorb and digest an adequate amount of nutrients on a temporary basis (Dougherty and Lamb, 1999)
⌘ Long-term nutritional support (Pennington et al, 1996)
⌘ If complete bowel rest is required
⌘ Patients with a short bowel, where the intestine is <200 cm.

Pre-procedure

Equipment required

⌘ Dressing trolley
⌘ Parenteral nutrition fluid and prescription chart
⌘ Giving set appropriate to the infusion pump being used
⌘ Infusion pump attached to a drip stand
⌘ Sterile dressing pack
⌘ Sterile gloves
⌘ Alcohol handrub.

Specific patient preparation required

⌘ Undertake a nutritional assessment
⌘ Ensure there is appropriate venous access for parenteral nutrition.

During the procedure

⌘ It is important to check patient name, date of birth and prescription. This ensures that the correct patient will receive the correct feed (follow local policy/protocol)

⌘ Clean the trolley and assemble the equipment required

⌘ Switch the infusion pump off and turn the clamp of the giving set off

⌘ Remove the empty bag and giving set

⌘ Suspend the feed complete with light protection cover on the drip stand as light affects the stability of the feed

⌘ Put on sterile gloves and insert the giving set into the parenteral nutrition bag and attach to the feeding line

⌘ Prime the line to ensure there are no air bubbles present that could lead to an air embolism (this will depend on the infusion pump in use, therefore manufacturer's guidelines should be followed)

⌘ Connect the giving set to the patient's cannula using a strict aseptic technique

⌘ Once a firm connection between the giving set, feed and the patient's feeding line has been established, a single layer of gauze may be wrapped around the hub connection and secured with tape with the end folded over (Bosonnet, 2002)

⌘ The giving set should then be inserted into the infusion pump, the volume and rate of infusion set according to prescription, and infusion commenced.

Post-procedure

⌘ Dispose of waste appropriately

⌘ Document the change of the bag on the prescription/order form and on the fluid balance chart

⌘ Observe for potential complications (*Box 6.8*)

Box 6.8: Potential complications of catheter line insertion

Pneumothorax	Post-subclavian catheterization, observe for chest pain and/or breathlessness
Haemorrhage	As a result of accidental arterial puncture of the carotid or subclavian arteries after central venous catheterization, observe site for signs of bleeding
Infection	Exit site infection, tunnel infection or catheter-related septicaemia – change the original dressing 24 hours post-procedure and then replace using an aseptic technique with an occlusive dressing that should be changed weekly unless the dressing becomes loose or wet (Tait, 2000; Field, 2002). A swab may need to be taken alongside blood cultures
Venous thrombosis	Caused by the catheter tip being situated high in the vena cava or subclavian vein. A venogram may be required for diagnostic purposes
Catheter occlusion	Check that the tip of the catheter is not kinked or twisted and ensure that medication is correctly administered, as well as fastidious aspiration

⌘ Flush the line with heparinized saline as prescribed to maintain patency

⌘ Record 4-hourly TPR to detect early signs of catheter-related sepsis, fluid overload or wound infection

⌘ Accurate recording of fluid balance is essential so that the patient's nutritional and fluid requirements can be estimated for the following day (Tait, 2000)

⌘ Weigh the patient daily to provide a more accurate measure of fluid balance (Daffurn et al, 1994)

⌘ Mouth care — often the patient is nil by mouth

⌘ Check capillary blood glucose every 4 hours for the initial 72 hours post-procedure, then twice-daily if stable. If the blood glucose is consistently higher than 12 mmol/l, sliding-scale insulin may be considered (Pennington, 2000)

⌘ Line entry and dressing sites should be checked and observed for warmth, redness, swelling and pain, which would indicate an infection (Hamilton, 2000)

⌘ Blood tests for biochemical analysis — this will enable the fluid and electrolyte balance, clinical condition and nutritional outcome to be monitored.

Rectal lavage

Rectal lavage is the washing out of the rectum using tap water or other recommended solutions. Local and national policy should be followed for the management of patients with functional bowel disorder (Royal College of Nursing (RCN), 2003; Gardiner et al, 2004). Rectal lavage is contraindicated for a number of reasons, including patients with haemorrhoids, anal fistulae, inflammatory bowel disease, rectal tumours, recent bowel surgery, heart failure and renal impairment. The rationale for the first five issues is the potential to mechanical damage; patients with heart failure and renal impairment are at risk from the potential to absorb fluid from the rectum during the procedure.

Reasons for the procedure

⌘ Before an investigation that requires the rectum to be clear of faeces

⌘ To prepare the rectum for surgery, decreasing the risk of infection

⌘ To clear the rectum of faeces for patients with functional bowel disorder secondary to a variety of diseases/disorders such as multiple sclerosis or spinal injury.

Pre-procedure

Equipment required

⌘ Incontinence sheet to protect bed linen

⌘ Non-sterile gloves and plastic aprons to protect from the potential risk of accidental spillage of faecal matter on the nurse's uniform

- Water-based lubrication jelly to lubricate the rectal tube for insertion
- Rectal tube — usually a specific rectal lavage catheter. Average length is up to 30 cm and width is usually 24 Fg
- Funnel, connector and tubing to connect to the rectal catheter
- Clamp to allow the rectal lavage catheter and tubing to be primed with water
- Jugs to contain tap water
- Tap water at a tepid temperature to prevent shock/discomfort of cold water being inserted into the rectum
- Bucket or large receiver to collect fluid after drainage from the rectum
- Wipes, soap and towel to clean the patient post-procedure
- Waste-disposal sack — biohazard.

Specific patient preparation required

- Clinical observations of pulse, respirations, blood pressure and peripheral saturations are recorded to act as a baseline to assess changes in the patient's condition
- The patient needs to remove clothes from the lower half of the body. Ensure the patient is comfortable lying in the left lateral position with knees drawn up towards the chest
- Protect the bed linen with incontinence sheets placed under the patient.

During the procedure

- Ensure that protective clothing is worn
- The rectal lavage tubing, funnel and connector are assembled and attached to the rectal catheter
- The set is primed with water to prevent insertion of air into the patient's rectum causing discomfort. The tubing is then clamped
- The patient's lower half of the body is exposed
- Ask the patient to try and relax, taking deep breaths to relax the anal sphincter
- A digital examination of the rectum is undertaken to ensure that the rectal catheter will pass easily and there are no obvious obstructions
- The rectal catheter is lubricated and inserted into the patient's rectum up to 10 cm in length
- Tepid tap water is inserted into the rectum via the funnel and rectal tubing, usually about 400 ml at a time. Gravity is used to feed the water into the rectum, with the funnel held approximately 30–50 cm above the patient's rectum
- Before the funnel has completely drained the water, the funnel is dropped down and inverted over the receiver or bucket. This is repeated until the waste fluid runs clear. No more than 6 litres of fluid is used during the lavage to reduce the potential risk of absorption of an excessive amount of water
- The amount of fluid used should be noted. The rectal tubing is removed and checked to see that it is complete and intact. The patient is assisted to use the toilet.

Post-procedure

⌘ Assist the patient to maintain his/her hygiene needs and to dress post-procedure
⌘ Have the call bell to hand so that the patient may summon assistance if required
⌘ Make a note of the amount of fluid used for the rectal lavage and compare this to the amount of effluent
⌘ Note the quantity, consistency and colour of faeces removed in the patient's notes
⌘ Record clinical observations to assess for any change in the patient's condition
⌘ Monitor for possible complications (*Box 6.9*).

Box 6.9: Complications of rectal lavage

Abdominal pain/cramping, secondary to evacuation of rectal matter

Perforation of the rectum

Damage to the anal sphincter

Water intoxication caused by absorption of water from the rectum

---

Collecting a stool specimen

The collection of a stool specimen is a non-invasive investigation that enables faecal matter to be examined in a pathology/microbiology department.

Reasons for the procedure

⌘ To detect abnormal pathogens
⌘ To detect occult blood
⌘ To aid diagnosis in malabsorption/inflammatory disorders/ malignancy.

Pre-procedure

Equipment required

⌘ Bedpan
⌘ Tissues
⌘ Stool chart

⌘ Pre-labelled sample container
⌘ Apron
⌘ Gloves
⌘ Sample request form.

Specific patient preparation required

⌘ Ensure privacy
⌘ Where possible help patient mobilize to the toilet. If unable, the patient may be able to use a commode or bedpan.

During the procedure

⌘ Ask patient to pass stool in clean container
⌘ Assist the patient with his/her hygiene needs
⌘ Examine stool (*Box 6.10*)

Box 6.10: Appearance of stool	
Black tarry stool	Bleeding high in the upper gastrointestinal tract
Maroon stool	Bleeding from the lower gastrointestinal tract
Fresh, bright blood	Problems in the anal canal
Putty-coloured stool	Obstruction to the flow of bile
From Gill (1999)	

⌘ Unscrew top of sample container, which has a small, plastic spade incorporated into the lid
⌘ Use the spade to place a small amount of faeces in the container and close the lid
⌘ Remove apron and gloves, and then wash hands.

Post-procedure

⌘ Date and time the collection of the sample on the container and the laboratory request form
⌘ Document collection of specimen in patient's notes and enter findings onto a stool chart if in use
⌘ Forward to appropriate laboratory following local policy.

Student skill laboratory activity
⌘ Identify the equipment required to undertake the collection of a stool specimen.

References

Arslantas A, Durmaz R, Cosan E, Tel E (2001) Inadvertent insertion of a nasogastric tube in a patient with head trauma. *Childs Nerv Syst* **17**(1–2): 112–14

ASPEN (2002) Guidelines for the use of enteral and parenteral nutrition in adult and paediatric patients. *J Parenter Enteral Nutr* 26(Suppl 1): 1SA–138SA

Bosonnet L (2002) Total parenteral nutrition: how to reduce the risks. *Nurs Times* **98**(22): 40–3

Daffurn K, Hillman KM, Bauman A, Lum M, Crispin C, Ince L (1994) Fluid balance charts: do they add up? *Br J Nurs* **3**: 816–20

Dougherty L, Lamb J (1999) *Intravenous Therapy in Nursing Practice*. Churchill Livingstone, London

Duncan HD, Silk DB (2001) Problems of treatment: enteral nutrition. In: Nightingale J, ed. *Intestinal Failure*. Greenwich Medical Media, London: 477–96

Evans D, Evans C, Evans R (2003) *The Procedure and Meaning of the Commoner Tests in Hospital*. 15th edn. Mosby, London

Field J (2002) Prevention of infection: central venous catheters. *Nurs Stand* **16**(38): 40–4

Gardiner A, Marshall J, Duthie G (2004) Rectal irrigation for relief of functional bowel disorders. *Nurs Stand* **10**(19): 39–42

Gill D (1999) Stool specimen. 1. Assessment. *Nurs Times* **95**(25): suppl 1–2

Hamilton H (2000) *Total Parenteral Nutrition: A Practical Guide for Nurses*. Churchill Livingstone, London

Holmes SA (2002) Nutrition and cancer. *Nurs Stand* **12**(5): 34–9

Littlejohn C (2004) Management of intentional overdose in A&E departments. *Nurs Times* **100**(33): 38–43

Lynch R, Robertson R (2003) Activated charcoal: the untold story. *Accid Emerg Nurs* **11**(2): 63–7

MacPhail J (2003) Irrigation technique. In: Elcoat C. *Stoma Care Nursing*. Bailliere Tindall, London

McConnell EA (1997) Inserting a nasogastric tube. *Nursing* **27**(1): 72

Metheny NA, Clouse RE, Clark JM, Reed L, Wehrle MA, Wiersema L (1994) pH testing of feeding-tube aspirates to determine placement. *Nutr Clin Pract* **9**: 185–90

Nursing and Midwifery Council (2002) *Code of Conduct*. NMC, London

Pennington CR (2000) What is parenteral nutrition? In: Hamilton H, ed. *Total Parenteral Nutrition: A Practical Guide for Nurses*. Churchill Livingstone, London

Pennington CR, Fawcett H, Macfie J, McWhirter J, Sizer T, Whithey S (1996) *Current Perspectives on Parenteral Nutrition in Adults*. BAPEN, Maidenhead

Royal College of Nursing (2003) *Digital Rectal Examination and Manual Removal of Faeces*. RCN, London

Smeltzer S, Bare B (eds) (2000) *Brunner and Suddarth's Textbook of Medical–Surgical Nursing*. 9th edn. Lippincott, Philadelphia

Smith G (2004) The management of acute upper gastrointestinal bleeding. *Nurs Times* **100**(26): 40–3

Stroud M, Duncan H, Nightingale J (2003) Guidelines for enteral feeding in adult hospital practice. *Gut* **52**(Suppl VII): vii1–vii2

Tait J (2000) Nursing management of the patient undergoing parenteral nutrition. In: Hamilton H, ed. *Total Parenteral Nutrition: A Practical Guide for Nurses*. Churchill Livingstone, London

Further reading

Abrams W, Beers M, Berkow M (1995) *Organ Systems; Gastrointestinal Disorders. The Merck Manual of Geriatrics*. Merck Research Labs, New Jersey, 7616–82

Alexander M, Fawcett J, Runciman P (eds) (2000) *Nursing Practice: Hospital and Home: the Adult*. 2nd edn. Churchill Livingstone, Edinburgh

Baker F, Smith L, Stead L, Soulsby C (1999) Inserting a nasogastric tube. *Nurs Times* **95**(7): suppl 1–2

Black PK (1994) Stoma care: a practical approach. *Nurs Stand* **8**(Suppl 34): 3–8

Burnham P (2000) A guide to nasogastric tube insertion. *NT Plus* **96**(8): 6–7

Cotton P, Williams C (1996) *Practical Gastrointestinal Endoscopy*. 4th edn. Blackwell Scientific, Oxford

Davenport R (2003) Preoperative stoma care. In: Elcoat C. *Stoma Care Nursing*. Bailliere Tindall, London

Devlin HB (1985) Living with a stoma. In: Devlin HB, ed. *Stoma Care Today*. Medical Education Services, Oxford, 34–7

Dougherty L, Lister S (eds) (2004) *The Royal Marsden Manual of Clinical Nursing Procedures*. 6th edn. Blackwell Scientific, Oxford

Evans D, Evans C, Evans R (2003) *The Procedure and Meaning of the Commoner Tests in Hospital*. 15th edn. Mosby, London

Heaton K, Radvan J, Cripps H, Mountford R, Braddon F, Hughes A (1992) Defaecation frequency and timing and stool form in the general population: a prospective study. *Gut* **33**: 181–24

Lawson A (2003) Complications of stomas. In: Elcoat C. *Stoma Care Nursing*. Bailliere Tindall, London

Metcalf C (1999) Stoma care: empowering patients through teaching practical skills. *Br J Nurs* **8**: 593–600

Nazarko L (1996) Preventing constipation in older people. *Prof Nurse* **11**: 816–18

Nursing and Midwifery Council (1992) *Scope of Professional Practice*. NMC, London

Nursing and Midwifery Council (1998) *Guidelines on Records and Record Keeping*. NMC, London

Nursing and Midwifery Council (2000) *Guidelines on the Administration of Drugs*. NMC, London

Nursing and Midwifery Council (2002) *Code of Conduct*. NMC, London

Readding L (2002) Stoma siting: what the community nurse needs to know. *Br J Community Nurs* **8**(11): 502–11

Royle J, Walsh M (1992) *Watsons Medical–Surgical Nursing and Related Physiology*. 4th edn. Bailliere Tindall, Eastbourne

Smith A, Lyon C, Hart C (2002) Multidisciplinary care of skin problems in stoma patients. *Br J Nurs* **11**: 324–30

Smith G (2004) Oesophageal varices. *Gastrointestinal Nursing* **2**(5): 33–8

Starr S, Hand H (2002) Nursing care of chronic and acute liver failure. *Nurs Stand* **16**(40): 47–54

Stuchfield B (2000) Stoma surgery in the older adults. *Elder Care* **11**(10): 49–56

Taylor P (2003) Clinical issues in stoma care practice. *Nursing and Residential Care* **5**(8): 366–70

Walsh M (ed) (2003) *Watson's Clinical Nursing and Related Sciences*. 6th edn. Bailliere Tindall, London

Williams J (2003) Types of stoma and associated surgical procedures. In: Elcoat C. *Stoma Care Nursing*. Bailliere Tindall, London

Useful websites

Alcohol Concern

www.alcoholconcern.org.uk

British Liver Trust

www.britishlivertrust.org.uk

British Society of Gastroenterology

www.bsg.org.uk

Chapter 7

Musculoskeletal and integumentary systems

Application of thromboembolic deterrent stockings

Thromboembolic deterrent stockings (TEDs) are a type of hosiery that when applied exerts sustained regressive pressure to the leg, with graduation decreasing from the ankle to the knee (Sigel et al, 1975). This mechanism promotes venous return and thus prevents venodilation, which subsequently causes microtears to the endothelium of the vein (Caprini et al, 1994). They are also known by other names such as graduated compression stockings (GCS) or anti-embolism stockings (AES). Deep vein thrombosis (DVT) is preventable (Autar, 1996; 2003); the application of TEDs reduces the risk of DVT by 68% (Wells et al, 1994). TEDs can be safely used with other forms of pharmacological prophylaxis such as heparin; when used as a combined regimen, DVT risk is reduced by 81% (Wille-Jorgensen et al, 1985).

Reasons for the procedure

⌘   Prophylactic management of DVT.

Pre-procedure

Equipment required

⌘   Tape measure
⌘   Pair of appropriately sized TED stockings
⌘   Applicator if recommended by hosiery manufacturer
⌘   Talcum powder.

Specific patient preparation required

⌘   Assess patient for potential contraindications (*Box 7.1*)
⌘   Explain the rationale for application of TED stockings in order to enhance compliance.

Box 7.1: Potential contraindications of TED hosiery

Venous ulceration causing broken skin

Known gangrenous condition of the limb

A recent skin graft

Advanced arteriosclerosis or peripheral vascular disease when Doppler pressure index is <0.8 (Scholten et al, 2000)

Cellulitis or dermatitis

Limb deformity making application difficult

Oversized thigh circumference for available TEDs

During procedure

- Expose limb(s) and measure accurately; TEDs are a medical device and need to be fitted precisely in order to achieve the clinically recognized compression profile
- All manufacturers provide their own measurement instructions
- To ease application of stocking, a small amount of talcum powder may be applied to the limb, or the stocking can be applied using an applicator
- Follow the step-by-step advice provided by the manufacturer for fitting the TED stocking
- Ill-fitting stockings can put patients at risk of DVT or of developing compression complications. Necrotic damage can be caused by compression (Callam et al, 1987; Merrett and Hanel, 1993)
- Ensure that any creases or wrinkles on the stockings are smoothed over
- Cover limb(s).

Post-procedure

- Inform the patient that TED stockings must be worn for 24 hours a day. They can be removed for short periods for skin inspection and hygiene. Stockings should not be left off for more than 30 minutes over the 24-hour period
- Stockings should be worn for as long as the patients are at high risk, as DVT can develop up to 6 weeks and beyond post-operatively (Scurr et al, 1988; Autar, 2002)
- Avoid skin lubrication with oily products as they may destroy the Lycra in the stockings
- Aqueous skin emollients or talcum powder are acceptable in moderation
- Stocking tops must not be turned down as this may have a tourniquet effect
- Most stockings are designed to stand up to about 30 washes. They can be washed every 2–3 days in order to prevent build up of body secretions, which can affect the elastic properties of the material. It is strongly recommended to follow the manufacturer's home laundry washing guide.

If hand washed, a mild detergent may be used with hand-hot water and the stockings should be allowed to dry naturally. After laundry, the stockings must be inspected for any holes or ladders in the fabric. If fabric is damaged, stockings must be renewed

⌘ Patients who are discharged home with TEDs should be supplied with at least two stockings — one to wear and the other for washing.

Student skill laboratory activity

⌘ Practise technique of limb measurement for the purpose of applying TED stockings

⌘ Apply TED stockings following manufacturer's guidelines.

Applying a plaster cast and cast management

A plaster cast is made up of plaster of paris bandages or synthetic materials. Plaster of paris is less frequently used, being replaced by fibreglass or lighter and sturdier materials. This procedure will focus on the application of plaster of paris and fibreglass casting.

Reasons for the procedure

⌘ To prevent and correct deformities
⌘ To provide support
⌘ To provide pain relief
⌘ To protect injury
⌘ To immobilize fractures
⌘ To improve function by stabilizing the joint
⌘ To permit early ambulation and weight bearing.

Pre-procedure

Equipment required

⌘ Plaster of paris
⌘ Stockinette if required
⌘ Plaster of paris slabs if required
⌘ Plaster strips to finish

- ⌘ Plastic sheeting and aprons
- ⌘ Plastic-covered pillows
- ⌘ Cast knife
- ⌘ Scissors
- ⌘ Bucket or bowl of water 20–25 °C
- ⌘ Wash bowl for patient
- ⌘ Towel(s)
- ⌘ Rubbish bag
- ⌘ Elbow or knee rest
- ⌘ Instruction leaflets
- ⌘ Synthetic padding and felt
- ⌘ Equipment trolley.

Specific patient preparation required

- ⌘ Any jewellery and clothing on the affected limb must be removed and stored safely by the patient or according to local policy
- ⌘ The prescription is checked for the correct details, and in readiness for undertaking the procedure an equipment trolley for the casting must be prepared
- ⌘ The patient is appropriately positioned for the limb to be casted. For upper limb casting, the patient is nursed in a supine position, with the shoulder abducted at 90°, elbow flexed at 90° and the digits held towards the ceiling. In lower-limb casting, the patient is positioned sitting up for a below-knee plaster of paris, and supine for a full-length or cylinder plaster. A footrest may be used to maintain the ankle in a neutral position during application.

During the procedure

Application of plaster of paris

- ⌘ A stockinette is applied for comfort, and protects the patient from the sharp edges of the plaster. It needs to be measured and cut a little longer than the plaster and then rolled up and applied to the limb. It is important to note that the application of stockinette will be contraindicated if there is likelihood of swelling as it may create a tourniquet effect and cause constriction
- ⌘ Bony prominences must be padded with synthetic felt for protection. This is followed by a layer of under-cast padding (wadding), applied smoothly and evenly over the stockinette, with any felt applied. The width of padding is usually 10–15 cm for lower extremity and 5–10 cm for upper extremity. The padding is applied by rolling distally to proximally, tearing it off to go around joints
- ⌘ Appropriate-sized plaster is selected for casting — 8–10 cm plaster is used for upper limb and 10–15 cm for lower limb
- ⌘ The plaster roll is prepared by unrolling the first 5–8 cm; keeping hold of the end it is then immersed into the container of lukewarm water (20–25 °C) until the bubbles stop. Cold water retards the setting process while warm water quickens it. With one end in each hand, the roll is gently squeezed to get rid of excess water

⌘ Bandaging commences at one end of the cast, rolling away from its applicator. The bandage is applied evenly, covering about one-third of the previous turn

⌘ The remainder of the bandages are then applied quickly before the first bandage is set

⌘ During the application process the palms of the hands and thenar eminences, rather than the fingertips, are used to constantly smooth and mould in order to fuse the bandages into one

⌘ It is important that the limb position is maintained throughout the application, therefore an additional nurse may be required to assist

⌘ After application the limb is rested on a pillow to prevent the cast from denting. Plastic or rubber pillows should not be used as they trap heat under the cast, which prevents heat dissipation and prolongs cast drying

⌘ The edges of the cast are trimmed and the proximal and distal ends of the stockinette are turned back over the cast edges, making a neat finish to prevent discomfort or injury.

Application of fibreglass cast

⌘ Fibreglass casts are becoming increasingly popular because they are durable, lightweight and waterproof. However, fibreglass is difficult to mould and significantly more expensive than plaster of paris, and is less used for acute injury, requiring frequent cast changes

⌘ The preparation of the patient is as for the application of plaster of paris. The procedure is similar to the application of plaster of paris described, except that:
  – wearing gloves is mandatory for handling the fibreglass material
  – a nylon stockinette and padding should be used
  – the roll of casting should be opened immediately before using

⌘ Fibreglass material must be applied with a little more pressure than plaster of paris, and conforms more easily if applied spirally, squaring the upper and lower ends by making horizontal turns

⌘ The cast needs to be applied so as to decrease the amount of trimming needed as fibreglass casts cannot be cut by the cast knife

⌘ After application the cast takes approximately 7 minutes to dry by the open-air drying method, and weight bearing is only allowed after 20 minutes.

Post-procedure

⌘ Elevate as appropriate, especially if swollen after activity

⌘ Allow to dry naturally at room temperature and leave uncovered for 48 hours. Drying times will vary and depend on the thickness of the plaster cast. As a rule, for regular, non-weight-bearing plaster casts the drying time is 24 hours; for weight-bearing plaster casts the drying time is 24–48 hours. The patient is allowed to bear weight after an X-ray shows reduction and immobilization of the fracture

⌘ Exercise joints not encased in plaster

⌘ In consultation with medical staff, clarify if the patient is allowed to weight bear on the cast

⌘ If cast edges become rough, cover the rough ends with tape

⌘ Wash the skin area around the cast, taking care not to wet the cast

⌘ Monitor for cracking, denting or softening of cast, swelling, discolouration, soreness, pins and needles, unpleasant smells, discharges and undue or increasing pain, and report to medical staff.

Student skills laboratory activity

⌘ Identify the equipment required for the application of a plaster cast

⌘ Practise applying a plaster cast on a suitable manikin.

Multi-layer compression bandaging

The use of external, graduated compression therapy that consists of the application of compression bandaging in the treatment of leg ulcers has been acknowledged as a recognized practice over the past decade (Rycroft-Malone, 2002). Before commencing compression therapy it is essential that the cause is correctly diagnosed, because inappropriate application of pressure to an ischaemic limb or arterial ulcer may have serious consequences by further impeding the already deficient blood supply. The diagnosis will be assisted by measurement of the ankle brachial pressure index (ABPI) (*Box 7.2*) using a Doppler ultrasound (Jones, 2000). Duplex scanning, which uses non-invasive imaging and blood flow measuring, may also be a useful tool (Ruckley, 1998).

Box 7.2: Ankle brachial pressure index (ABPI)

$$\frac{\text{Ankle systolic blood pressure}}{\text{Brachial systolic blood pressure}} = \textbf{ABPI}$$

The four-layer bandage system was developed to apply 40 mmHg pressure at the ankle, graduating to 17 mmHg pressure at the knee, using bandages of different properties. Several different bandaging systems are available, each of which may have advantages over the others for particular applications.

Multi-layer bandaging should provide adequate padding, adequate compression and sustained compression for at least a week at a time, and should provide comfort and ease of use.

Patients with arterial disorders or microvascular disease may not be considered suitable for compression therapy.

Reasons for the procedure

⌘ Increase blood velocity in the deep veins
⌘ Reduce oedema and therefore reduce the pressure differential between the capillaries and the tissues
⌘ Reduce distension of superficial veins and reverse venous hypertension
⌘ Improve the healing rate of chronic venous ulcers
⌘ Comfort and ease of use to ensure patient concordance.

Pre-procedure

Equipment required

⌘ Prescribed wound dressing to facilitate healing of the wound bed
⌘ Warm normal saline solution (0.9%) to irrigate wound
⌘ Orthopaedic wool bandage (layer 1)
⌘ Cotton crepe bandage 10 cm wide (layer 2)
⌘ Light-compression bandage 10 cm wide that provides 14–17 mmHg pressure (layer 3)
⌘ Moderate-compression cohesive bandage 10 cm wide that provides 17–23 mmHg pressure (layer 4)
⌘ Adhesive tape
⌘ Emollient cream
⌘ Facilities to wash and dry the foot and leg
⌘ Non-sterile gloves and apron
⌘ Protection for the floor.

Specific patient preparation required

⌘ The patient may be seated during the procedure, or may be in a semi-reclined position on a bed
⌘ Manual handling issues are taken into consideration to avoid stooping and twisting
⌘ Consideration should also be given to the ability of the patient to elevate his/her leg for the procedure, and in some instances a second nurse may be required to hold the leg in position.

During the procedure

⌘ Apply non-sterile gloves and apron
⌘ Open dressing packs and bandages onto a clean, dry area
⌘ Remove old bandaging carefully and dispose as per local clinical waste policy. Washing bandages is not recommended as this may affect elasticity and thus subsequent pressure application (Eagle, 2001)
⌘ Wash leg around wound and dry well
⌘ Irrigate wound with warmed saline
⌘ Apply chosen wound dressing
⌘ Apply emollient to surrounding skin after ensuring patient compatibility
⌘ Apply orthopaedic wool bandage (layer 1) as a layer of padding, paying particular attention to prominences such as shin, malleoli and achilles areas
⌘ Apply crepe bandage (layer 2) in a spiral as a retaining layer from base of toes to below the knee and secure with tape
⌘ Apply light-compression bandage (layer 3) in a figure of eight from base of toes to below the knee and secure with tape. This layer can be omitted if three-layer bandaging is advocated
⌘ Apply moderate-compression cohesive bandage (layer 4) in spiral from base of toes to below knee and secure with tape.

Post-procedure

⌘ Check for comfort and reassure patient

⌘ Check toes for colour, warmth, movement and sensitivity to monitor circulation

⌘ Document procedure, evaluate healing and report signs of wound deterioration and review wound management strategy as necessary

⌘ Give advice and education to patient on the care of the bandaging (*Box 7.3*) to prevent infection and other complications

---

Box 7.3: Advice to patients on how to care for bandages

Keep bandages dry

Avoid tight-fitting footwear that might further compress the toes

Contact nurse if bandages ride down the leg as this can cause pre-tibial skin necrosis

Contact nurse if excessive exudate staining is evident on top layer, which might indicate the need for bandage change to avoid skin excoriation

It is recommended that bandages remain unchanged for 1 week to sustain the pressure obtained by compression

---

⌘ Dispose of equipment and wash hands.

Student skill laboratory activity

⌘ Assemble all the equipment you would require to undertake compression therapy

⌘ Practise applying four-layer bandaging on a manikin.

Skin closure

Skin closure is the alignment and bringing together of skin edges to facilitate optimal healing. Skin closure comprises a number of methods: suturing, stapling, gluing, hair tying and the use of adhesive closure strips. The method of skin closure depends on the nature of the wound:

⌘ *Sutures.* Suture material is either absorbable or non-absorbable:
  —absorbable sutures such as catgut or vicryl take around 4 wecks to dissolve, thus are most useful for internal and deeper wounds (Cole, 2003)

—non-absorbable sutures such as nylon, polypropylene or silk are most suitable for wounds of the dermis and epidermis.
Suture thickness is measured by gauge, with 6.0 being the smallest and 3.0 the thickest

⌘ *Staples*. These are disposable single-use packs and are applied by a surgical stapler (Richardson, 2003). The superficial wound edges need to be in alignment for staples to be effective. McClelland and Nellis (1997) suggest that stainless steel staples provide an environment non-conducive to bacterial growth, which is particularly important when wounds are contaminated from the original source of the wound

⌘ *Glue*. Glue is often used as an alternative to suturing for simple, dry lacerations. It works through polymerization and achieves a good cosmetic result (Farion, 2003). Charters (2000) identified glue to be most successful on scalp lacerations

⌘ *Adhesive closure strips*. These are available in a wide variety of lengths and widths. They can be used in conjunction with staples and sutures to provide additional support. Used on their own, adhesive closure strips do not require local anaesthetic for application. They are most commonly used for simple, superficial lacerations. Adhesive closure strips cannot be used for deep wounds or be applied to hairy, oily skin surfaces (Gottrup, 1999)

⌘ *Hair ties*. This closure method is only suitable for simple scalp lacerations that are not actively bleeding.

Reasons for the procedure

⌘ To support the damaged tissues while healing occurs
⌘ To minimize the risk of developing a localized infection and reduce the risk of future bleeding
⌘ To provide a visually aesthetic result.

Pre-procedure

Equipment required

⌘ Appropriate closure equipment
⌘ 0.9% normal saline (warmed)
⌘ 50 ml syringe
⌘ 19-gauge needle
⌘ Dressing pack
⌘ Additional dressings to cover wound as required
⌘ Gloves
⌘ Goggles (or other protective eye equipment)
⌘ Lidocaine hydrochloride
⌘ Sterile forceps
⌘ Sharps bin.

Specific patient preparation required

⌘ Undertake a comprehensive wound assessment (*Box 7.4*) to identify the skin closure method to be used and the material required

---

Box 7.4: Factors to be considered in a wound assessment

Establish the cause of injury/wound

Duration of the wound

Depth of wound

Site of wound

Tissue type involved

Presence of infection

Pain

Measuring wound

Wound edge

Condition of surrounding skin

⌘ The wound should be appropriately cleansed and debrided if required. To remove the debris from the wound, high-pressure irrigation using a 50 ml syringe and a 19-gauge needle is most effective (Richardson, 2004). This provides 4–15 psi (pounds per square inch) and safely removes contamination from the wound without causing further damage (Bergstrom, 1994)

⌘ The wound should be infiltrated with a prescribed local anaesthetic, such as lidocaine hydrochloride (British Medical Association and Royal Pharmaceutical Society of Great Britain, 2003).

During the procedure

Adhesive closure strips

⌘ The correctly sized closure strips are selected for the wound — the strip must cover the diameter of the wound and have a clean and dry area at either side for it to securely adhere to. Strips are available in 3 mm, 6 mm and 12 mm sizes

⌘ Starting at the middle of the wound, the first closure strip is applied by apposing the wound edges together. This can either be achieved by using forceps or a sterile, gloved finger depending on where the wound is located

⌘ Starting in the middle and applying other strips towards the outward edge of the wound will maintain skin position and prevent the wound healing in a displaced manner. Careful wound edge alignment will ensure a good cosmetic result

⌘ The strips should ideally be 3 mm apart (Richardson, 2003) to allow draining of any exudates or bleeding.

Suturing technique

⌘ Nurses should not attempt to suture unless they are competent to do so

⌘ The suture needle is held in a pair of forceps and is inserted about 5 mm from one skin edge, which is itself held and supported with more forceps. The suture is pulled through into the open wound

⌘ The needle is next inserted separately through the open wound and should exit through the skin on the opposite side of the wound, about 5 mm from the edge

⌘ Skin edges should be slightly elevated during this procedure to aid wound healing. The suture is knotted on one side of the wound line. If sutures are tied too tightly, tissues can become damaged; while sutures tied too loosely fail to hold tissues in adequate apposition and may result in delayed healing and in scar lines that are cosmetically unacceptable.

Hair tying

⌘ This involves taking hair from both sides of a scalp wound and tying it across the wound to achieve tissue apposition. This can be achieved through a series of evenly spaced hair knots for a secure closure line

⌘ The knots can be further fixed with tissue adhesive (Aoki, 1996).

Gluing

⌘ The glue vial is squeezed gently either to spread a thin line of adhesive along the length of the wound or to 'spot weld' the wound closed by applying a series of dots along its length

⌘ The wound needs to be held together for 30 seconds to allow polymerization.

Staples

⌘ To insert staples the wound edges need to be carefully apposed and if possible elevated slightly to avoid scar deformity. The stapler is then placed gently across the wound and the handle squeezed to release the staple

⌘ Excessive pressure on the skin should be avoided as this can give poor cosmetic results and make staple removal difficult.

Post-procedure

⌘ Dispose of equipment as per local policy

⌘ Correct documentation of the closure procedure

⌘ Ascertain the patient's tetanus status in accordance with the Department of Health (2002) recommendations for immunizations

⌘ Apply additional dressing if required.

Student skill laboratory activity

⌘ Assemble equipment required for skin closure and practise skin closure on appropriate manikin.

Removal of skin closure material

The main principle behind suture removal is to ensure that no part of the suture that is visible above the skin should be drawn underneath the skin, to prevent infection developing in the healing wound tissue (Workman and Bennett, 2003). The principle behind all wound closure material is to hold the wound edges in apposition to promote effective and timely wound healing, to produce minimal scar tissue and to prevent wound infection.

Sutures and staples are removed after 3–10 days depending on the site and type of the wound (Wyatt, 2003). Adhesive closure strips can remain in place for 5–7 days for simple lacerations (Cole, 2003). If strips lose their adhesiveness before the wound-healing process has completed, more strips can be applied over the top of the existing strips to secure the wound for a longer period of time. When ready, they are simply removed by peeling off alternate strips from the wound — warmed 0.9% sodium chloride solution may reduce their adhesiveness. Hair ties do not need to be removed unless they cause irritation, otherwise they will grow out as the surrounding hair grows.

Reasons for the procedure

⌘ When the wound has healed. Delayed removal initiates the body to respond as though a foreign object remains within the scar tissue, which may result in further scarring.

Pre-procedure

Equipment required

⌘ Equipment as for aseptic technique including sterile dressing pack with forceps and gloves

⌘ Sterile stitch cutter, sterile scissors or staple/clip remover, according to the wound closure material

⌘ Normal saline

⌘ Suitable dressing if necessary

⌘ Sharps container.

Specific patient preparation required

- Establish whether all or interrupted sutures are to be removed
- Position the patient to expose the wound site
- If dressings are present, loosen and remove following standard precautions
- Examine the wound and skin integrity before removing the sutures. The wound should show signs of healing. Excessive wound inflammation or discharge should be reported to the nurse in charge before proceeding, as a wound swab may be required and only alternative sutures removed on this occasion
- Establish the number of sutures/staples to be removed
- When removing any type of wound-closure devices, inform the patient that they may feel slight discomfort, such as a pulling or stinging sensation. Moisten dried crusts with warmed 0.9% sodium chloride solution, wearing clean gloves.

During the procedure

Individual or interrupted sutures

- Hold the knot with sterile forceps and slightly lift it away from the surface of the skin
- Slide the stitch cutter or scissor tips under the suture opposite to the knot and as close to the skin surface as possible and cut the suture here (*Figure 7.1*)
- The suture is pulled upwards from the knot end. Use the tips of the scissors held slightly apart or the edge of the blade cutter to gently press on the skin when the suture is drawn out, to ease its withdrawal and lessen the resistance from the skin

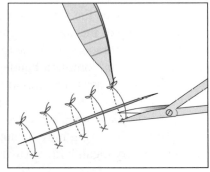

Figure 7.1: Individual or interrupted suture removal

- Place removed sutures on some gauze
- If the wound is longer than 15 cm, remove alternate sutures first to determine wound integrity. If healing has taken place sufficiently then all the sutures can be removed (Nicol et al, 2003; Workman and Bennett, 2003)
- Count and discard the sutures
- If necessary, clean the wound site with normal saline and place a suitable dressing over the suture line if the patient wishes, for his/her comfort (Workman and Bennett, 2003).

Continuous suture line

- Cut the first suture at the end furthest from the knot
- Use the forceps to lift the next suture and loosen it from the skin. It is imperative that only one end of the suture is cut to ensure complete removal of the entire suture (*Figure 7.2*). The exposed part of the suture should not be pulled through the tissues

❋ Repeat this process along the suture line, until all portions have been removed

❋ If any part of the wound edge appears to be gaping, skin-closure strips can be applied to assist the healing process

❋ A suitable dressing may be applied and the wound site cleaned as necessary.

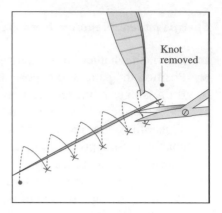

Knot removed

Figure 7.2: Continuous suture line removal

Removal of staples/clips

❋ The specific staple or clip removal tool is used here. It is designed to fit under the centre of the staple, and slight pressure causes the ends of the staple to lift out of the skin

❋ Slide the lower jaw of the staple remover under the centre of the first staple and keep it close to the skin

❋ The upper jaw rests above the top of the staple. Squeezing the handles of the remover together will close the jaws so that the top of the staple is depressed and the prongs will lift out of the intradermal tissue (*Figure 7.3*)

❋ Place the non-dominant hand gently either side of the staple during this process to support the skin and prevent pulling

❋ Lift the staples out and place on gauze. Count to ensure that all staples have been removed

❋ A suitable dressing may be applied over the wound site and if necessary clean with normal saline.

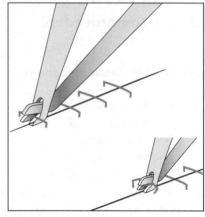

Figure 7.3: Staple removal

Post-procedure

❋ Dispose of equipment as appropriate, ensuring that sharp objects such as stitch cutters are disposed of in the sharps bin

❋ Document removal of suture material in the nursing records, reporting on the status of the wound and any changes to the planned intervention.

Student skill laboratory activity

❋ Identify the equipment you would require to remove sutures and staples

❋ Practise removing sutures and staples from a suitable manikin.

Traction

Traction means the drawing of an injured or diseased part of the body along a plane. In order to pull an object in one direction, there must be an equal force or counterthrust in the opposite direction. There are two main types of traction — fixed and sliding:

⌘ *Fixed traction.* This is the traction between two fixed points, as in a Thomas' splint (*Figure 7.4*). The two fixed points are the force applied to the pull of the extension cords tied to the end of the splint, and the force that is transmitted along the parallel bars pushing against the ischial tuberosity

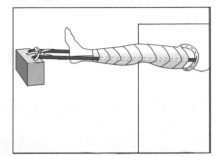

Figure 7.4: A fixed traction

⌘ *Sliding traction.* This is also known as balanced traction. In sliding traction there must be two opposing forces, this time balanced and each of comparable weight. In sliding traction, the bed is tilted so that the patient tends to slide or move in the opposite direction to that of the traction force. The balance is the traction from the limb by the weights, and the counter traction is the patient's own weight sliding in the opposite direction (*Figure 7.5*).

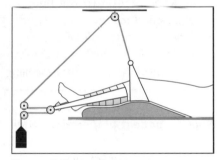

Figure 7.5: A sliding traction

Reasons for the procedure

⌘ To reduce dislocation or fracture
⌘ To prevent movement of injured part, thus facilitating bone healing
⌘ To reduce and overcome muscle spasm
⌘ To prevent and correct deformity
⌘ To rest joints
⌘ To allow healing in the optimum position.

Pre-procedure

Equipment required for the application of Thomas' splint

⌘ Skin preparation material as required
⌘ Skin extension or pinholder for skeletal traction

⌘ 15 cm calico slings cut to the appropriate size
⌘ Gamgee for comfort
⌘ Crepe bandages and adhesive strapping
⌘ Scissors
⌘ Pearson knee flexion piece
⌘ Traction cord
⌘ Three pulleys — two for the overhead bar and one on the frame at the front of the bed
⌘ Weights
⌘ Suspension system
⌘ Safety pins for securing calico slings
⌘ Thomas' splint as required (*Box 7.5*).

Box 7.5: Selection and measurement of Thomas' splint

In order to determine the correct ring size, the level of the greater trochanter to the adductor tendon in the groin is measured. The length of the splint is measured from the adductor tendon to the heel plus 30 cm to allow for the extension bow. The splint must also be supplied for specific left or right leg. The ring is set obliquely at an angle of 120° to the medial bar; one-half of the ring is slightly larger than the other half to take the posterior portion of the thigh and the hamstring muscle. A half or split ring is preferred in order to accommodate any initial swelling

---

Specific patient preparation required

⌘ Shaving as necessary
⌘ Position and alignment
⌘ Pain relief
⌘ Care of the skin around the ring of the Thomas' splint
⌘ Expose the affected limb and remove clothing.

During the procedure

⌘ The splint is prepared by using calico slings and safety pins to create a cradle along the length of the Thomas' splint for supporting the limb
⌘ A layer of gamgee is placed along most of the length of the sling, stopping at the heel
⌘ The splint should be positioned to create 5° of knee flexion. This can be achieved by placing additional gamgee in the knee region. If more than 5° of knee flexion is required, a Pearson knee flexion piece is used. This is attached to the parallel bars of the splint
⌘ The skin or skeletal traction is then applied and the prepared splint passed over the limb
⌘ The splint is pushed up to the groin and the tension of the slings adjusted to maintain normal bowing of the femur

⌘ At the w-shaped distal end of the splint, the skin extension cords, if applied, are tied to the end of the splint with sufficient force to prevent the splint ring from embedding in the groin (Stewart and Hallett, 1983)

⌘ Crepe bandages are applied above and below the knee to keep the extensions in place over the limb and are secured with adhesive strapping. More bandages may be applied over the lateral and medial bars of the splint

⌘ In this way the traction is achieved by the pull on the extension, and the foot of the bed is elevated for counter traction

⌘ After application of the traction, the suspension system is set up to facilitate the mobility of the patient while being maintained on the Thomas' splint.

Post-procedure

⌘ Undue pressure in the popliteal space must be prevented by ensuring that the sling is well padded, crease-free and the pillow is not hard

⌘ Patients must be taught to lift their buttock off the bed frequently by using the overhead trapeze and their unaffected leg, so as to reduce risk of sacral tissue damage. Foot exercises must be encouraged regularly to the affected foot to maintain strength and prevent footdrop

⌘ The knee should be left exposed

⌘ Ensure good skin care

⌘ Liaise with the physiotherapist regarding exercise education.

Hamilton Russell traction

This type of traction is primarily used preoperatively to overcome muscular spasm and pain in patients with fractured neck of femur.

Equipment

⌘ Skin preparation material as required
⌘ Below-knee skin extension
⌘ Padded knee sling
⌘ Crepe bandages to apply over extensions (15 cm)
⌘ Adhesive strapping to secure bandage
⌘ Scissors
⌘ Traction cord
⌘ Three pulleys — one over the knee and two at the end of the bed
⌘ Soft pillow to support the leg
⌘ Weights as prescribed.

Specific patient preparation required: application

❈ A below-knee skin extension is applied and the leg is supported on a soft pillow with the knee flexed, leaving the heel clear of pressure

❈ A padded sling passes around the knee, to which the traction cord is tied and sited vertically onto a mounted pulley on the overhead frame

❈ A spreader is applied to the footplate of the skin extension to allow for a horizontal pull via a two-pulley system (*Figure 7.6*)

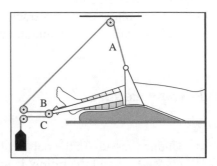

Figure 7.6: Traction using vectored forces

❈ Two forces are used to maintain the desired traction. A vertical pull is exerted on the leg through the sling under the knee, while the horizontal pull is achieved using the two pulleys at the footplate of the skin extension. This pulley arrangement, whereby the traction goes from a patient to a frame and then back to the patient, creates a vectored force (Taylor, 1987) — the horizontal pull to an extremity is double the amount of weight applied

❈ The two combined weights produce the resultant pull

❈ The foot of the bed is elevated to provide counter traction.

Post-procedure

❈ The patient should be nursed on a firm-based bed for full support and to allow for efficient action of the traction system

❈ The traction should be checked a minimum of twice a day as the system may be inadvertently altered or interfered with during clinical procedures

❈ The traction cord should be checked for fraying, and the line of pull of the cord should also be regularly checked and corrected

❈ Pulleys must be free running and weights should hang freely and not rest on the floor

❈ In skeletal traction, pointed ends of the pins must be covered to prevent injury to the patient and staff

❈ Pin sites should be cared for aseptically and according to local protocol derived from evidence-based practice

❈ Ensure good skin care

❈ Liaise with the physiotherapist regarding exercise education.

References

Aoki N (1996) Hair braiding for superficial wounds. *Surg Neurol* **46**(2): 150–1

Autar R (1996) *Deep Vein Thrombosis: The Silent Killer*. Quay Books, Salisbury

Autar R (2002) *Advancing clinical practice in the management of deep vein thrombosis (DVT). Development, application and evaluation of the Autar DVT scale*. PhD dissertation. De Montfort University, Leicester

Autar R (2003) The management of deep vein thrombosis: the Autar DVT risk assessment scale revisited. *J Orthopaed Nurs* **7**(3): 114–24

Bergstrom N (1994) *Treatment of Pressure Ulcers*. Department of Health Care Policy Research, Nebraska, USA

British Medical Association and Royal Pharmaceutical Society of Great Britain (2003) *British National Formulary 45*. BMA/RPSGB, London

Callam MJ, Harper DR, Dale JJ, Ruckley CV (1987) Arterial disease in chronic leg ulceration: an underestimated hazard? Lothian and Firth Valley leg ulcer study. *Br Med J* **294**: 929–31

Caprini JA, Arcelus JI, Hoffman BA et al (1994) Prevention of venous thromboembolism in North America. Results of a survey among general surgeons. *J Vasc Surg* **20**(5): 751–7

Charters A (2000) Wound glue: a comparative study of tissue adhesives. *Accid Emerg Nurs* **8**: 223–7

Cole E (2003) Wound management in A&E department. *Nurs Stand* **17**(46): 45–52

Department of Health (2002) *The Green Book: Immunisation Against Infectious Disease*. DoH, London

Eagle M (2001) Compression bandaging. *Nurs Stand* **15**(38): 47–52

Farion K (2003) Tissue adhesives for traumatic lacerations: a systematic review of randomised controlled trials. *Acad Emerg Med* **10**(2): 110–18

Gottrup F (1999) Wound closure technique. *J Wound Care* **8**: 397–400

Jones J (2000) The use of holistic assessment in the treatment of leg ulcers. *Br J Nurs* **9**: 1040–52

McClelland H, Nellis G (1997) Surgical staple trial in Accident and Emergency. *Accid Emerg Nurs* **5**: 62–4

Merrett ND, Hanel KC (1993) Ischaemic complications of graduated compression stockings in the treatment of deep venous thrombosis. *Postgrad Med J* **69**(809): 232–4

Nicol M, Bavin C, Bedford-Turner S, Cronin P, Rawlings-Workman BA, Bennett CL (2003) *Key Nursing Skills*. Whurr Publishers, London: 293

Richardson M (2003) Wound closure. *Emerg Nurse* **11**(3): 25–32

Richardson M (2004) Procedures for cleansing, closing and covering acute wounds. *Nurs Times* **100**(4): 54–9

Ruckley CV (1998) Caring for patients with chronic leg ulcer. *Br Med J* **316**: 407–8

Rycroft-Malone J (2002) Getting evidence into practice: ingredients for change. *Nurs Stand* **16**(37): 38–43

Scholten P, Bever A, Turner K, Warburton L (2000) Graduated elastic compression stockings on a stroke unit: a feasibility study. *Age Ageing* **29**: 357–9

Scurr J, Coleridge-Smith PD, Hasty J (1988) Deep vein thrombosis: a continuing problem. *Br Med J* **297**: 28

Sigel B, Edelstein AL, Savitch L et al (1975) Type of compression for reducing venous stasis: a study of lower extremities during inactive recumbency. *Arch Surg* **110**: 171

Stewart JDM, Hallett JP (1983) *Traction and Orthopaedic Appliances*. 2nd edn. Churchill Livingstone, London

Taylor I (1987) *Ward Manual of Orthopaedic Traction*. Churchill Livingstone, Edinburgh

Wells P, Lensing A, Hirsch J (1994) Graduated compression stockings in the prevention of postoperative venous thromboembolism: a meta-analysis. *Arch Intern Med* **151:** 67–72

Wille-Jorgensen P, Throup J, Fisher A et al (1985) Heparin with and without graded compression stockings in the prevention of thromboembolic complications of major abdominal surgery: a randomised trial. *Br J Surg* **72:** 579–81

Workman BA, Bennett CL (2003) *Key Nursing Skills*. Whurr Publishers, London

Wyatt JP (2003) *Oxford Handbook of Accident and Emergency Medicine*. Oxford University Press, Oxford

Further reading

Anderson GH, Harper WM, Connolly CD et al (1993) Preoperative skin traction for fractures of the proximal femur: a randomised prospective trial. *J Bone Joint Surg* **75-B:** 794–6

Anderson K (2001) Essential skills. 18. Wound assessment. Removal of skin closures. *Nurs Stand* **16**(8): 2

Apley AG, Solomon L (1994) *Concise System of Orthopaedics and Fractures*. Butterworth Heinemann, Oxford

Carrington C (1999) A nurse-led clinic for managing venous leg ulcers. *Nurs Stand* **13**(20): 42–6

Cullum N, Roe B (1995) *Leg Ulcers: Nursing Management*. Scutari Press, Oxford

Dandy D (1993) *Essential Orthopaedics and Trauma*. 2nd edn. Churchill Livingstone, Edinburgh

Davies C (2001) Use of Doppler ultrasound in leg assessment. *Nurs Stand* **15**(44): 72–4

Davis PS (1994) *Nursing the Orthopaedic Patient*. Churchill Livingstone, Edinburgh

Davis P, Barr L (1999) Principles of traction. *J Orthopaed Nurs* **3:** 222–7

Laing W (1992) *Chronic Venous Diseases of the Leg*. Office of Health Economics, London

Mills K (1986) *Plastering Techniques*. Wolfe Medical, London

Moffatt CI (1992) Compression bandaging: the state of the art. *J Wound Care* **1**(1): 45–50

Moffatt C, Harper P (1997) *Access to Clinical Education: Leg Ulcers*. Churchill Livingstone, New York

Morgan S (1989) *Plaster Casting. Patients' Problems and Nursing Care*. Heinemann Nursing, Oxford

Pearson A (1987) *Living in a Plaster Cast*. RCN Series. Whitefriars Press, London

Prior M, Miles S (1999) Principles of casting. *J Orthopaed Nurs* **3:** 162–70

Pudner R (1997) Wound cleansing. *J Community Nurs* **11**(7): 30–6

Smith L, Baker F, Stead L (1999) Removal of sutures. Practical procedures for nurses Part 25.1. *Nurs Times* **95**(9): suppl 1–2

Smith L, Baker F, Stead L (1999) Removal of sutures. Practical procedures for nurses Part 25.2. *Nurs Times* **95**(10): suppl 1–2

Torrance C, Serginson E (1997) *Surgical Nursing*. 12th edn. Balliere Tindall, London

Chapter 8

Neurological system

Lumbar puncture

A lumbar puncture (LP) is an invasive procedure that involves the removal of cerebrospinal fluid (CSF) through a puncture into the subarachnoid space of the spinal cord. LP should be avoided if the patient demonstrates any of the following:

⌘ A raised intracranial pressure
⌘ Depressed consciousness
⌘ Concomitant coagulopathy
⌘ Tissue sepsis
⌘ Congenital abnormalities of the lumbar region (Bassett, 1997).

Reasons for the procedure

⌘ To aid diagnosis
⌘ To facilitate the administration of intrathecal medicine (Bassett, 1997; Blows, 2002).

Pre-procedure

Equipment required

⌘ Trolley
⌘ Lumbar puncture needle/spinal needle
⌘ Dressing pack
⌘ Antiseptic to clean the skin
⌘ 10 ml syringe
⌘ Various gauge needles
⌘ Local anaesthetic
⌘ Three sterile universal containers labelled 1, 2 and 3
⌘ Glucose blood bottles x 2
⌘ Phlebotomy equipment

* Manometer
* Three-way tap
* Small dressing (establish if the patient has any allergies)
* Sterile gloves
* Gloves.

Specific patient preparation required

* Offer the patient toilet facilities as necessary
* Establish a method of communication with the patient to indicate that he/she wishes to move
* Obtain a sample of venous blood 30–60 minutes before the procedure being undertaken and place this in a blood glucose bottle. This can then be compared with the CSF glucose level (Tate and Tasota, 2000)
* Position the patient as close to the edge of the bed as possible, for ease of access. The patient can be sitting up and bent over a table or lying on one side with his/her knees drawn up towards the chest and the back exposed. Such a position curves the spine, maximizes spaces between the vertebrae and facilitates entry of the lumbar puncture needle/spinal needle (Bassett, 1997; Tate and Tasota, 2000; Blows, 2002).

During the procedure

* Assist the doctor/practitioner in preparing for the aseptic procedure
* The lumbar puncture needle/spinal needle is introduced below the level of the spinal cord into the lumbar cisterna through the third lumbar vertebra (L3) or fourth lumbar vertebra (L4), passing via the dura and arachnoid maters into the subarachnoid space (*Figure 8.1*).

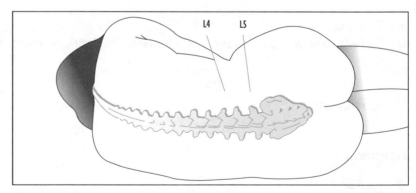

Figure 8.1: Positioning for lumbar puncture

* Support the patient to keep still to try and prevent any injury to the spinal cord
* A manometer will be attached to measure CSF pressure (60–160 mmH$_2$O), a raise in pressure being indicative of a raised ICP. In numerical order, three samples are collected as initially blood caused by trauma may contaminate the sample. The sample of CSF is taken for protein, glucose, lactate and lymphocytes (*Box 8.1*)

Box 8.1: Normal CSF values

Protein 15–45 mg per 100 ml

Glucose 40–80 mg per 100 ml

Lactate 1.1–1.9 mmol per litre

Lymphocytes 0–5 cells per mm^3

From Blows (2002)

⌘ Place a small dressing on the puncture site

⌘ Note the colour of the CSF; it is usually a watery, clear liquid. However, if the CSF is continuous fresh blood, this is indicative of very recent bleeding into the subarachnoid space. If the CSF is a continuous yellow stain (xanthochromia), this may be indicative of an older subarachnoid bleed.

Post-procedure

⌘ To prevent a headache from occurring as a consequence of removal of CSF, the patient should be advised to lay flat for 6–12 hours (Hickey, 1997). If there is no headache then the patient can resume normal activities

⌘ Analgesia should be given as prescribed and the effect evaluated

⌘ The dressing site should be checked for signs of leakage, bleeding or inflammation, and the dressing changed as required

⌘ Ensure that all CSF samples are secured, the bottle labelled and forwarded with the correct microbiology request form

⌘ Dispose of equipment

⌘ Record the date and time that the procedure was undertaken in the patient's documentation

⌘ The findings may indicate a number of medical conditions (*Box 8.2*).

Box 8.2: Changes related to medical conditions

Rise in protein	Infection of the meninges or brain, brain tumour or multiple sclerosis
Disturbance in lactate	Central nervous system infection
Lowered glucose	Bacterial infection
Increase in lymphocytes	Infection

From Bassett (1997); Blows (2002)

Neurological observations

The Glasgow Coma Scale (GCS) is an assessment tool that is often combined with the recording of vital signs under the umbrella term 'neurological observations'. The GCS consists of a set of observations that indicate how well the brain is functioning (Jennett and Teasdale, 1981). It is used in most neurological centres, and the National Institute for Clinical Excellence (2003) recommends that the GCS should be used to assess all brain-injured patients.

The GCS assesses two aspects of consciousness:

⌘ *Arousal*. Being aware of the environment
⌘ *Cognition*. Demonstrating an understanding of what the observer has said through an ability to perform tasks (Shah, 1999).

Each activity that the patient performs is given a score; the best score is 15 and the worst score is 3. A reduction in the score may reflect a deteriorating condition and should be urgently brought to the attention of the doctors in charge of the patient.

Reasons for the procedure

⌘ To monitor level of consciousness
⌘ To aid diagnosis
⌘ To indicate the effectiveness of treatment.

Pre-procedure

Equipment required

⌘ Neurological observation chart
⌘ Torch
⌘ Pen
⌘ Sphygmomanometer
⌘ Thermometer
⌘ Watch with a second hand.

Specific patient preparation required

⌘ Before undertaking the neurological assessment, it is important that the patient is maximally aroused to give an accurate result.

During the procedure

⌘ The practitioner applies the categories shown in *Box 8.3* in the assessment of eye opening, verbal response and motor response. These provide information about responses in the brain.

Box 8.3: Glasgow Coma Scale	
Eye opening	
Spontaneously	4
To speech	3
To pain	2
No response	1
Best verbal response	
Orientated	5
Confused	4
Inappropriate speech	3
Incomprehensible speech	2
No response	1
T = intubated/tracheostomy	
Best motor response	
Obeys commands	6
Localizes to pain	5
Flexes to pain	4
Abnormal flexion	3
Abnormal extension	2
No response	1
Lowest possible score = 3; highest possible score = 15. From Jennett and Teasdale (1974)	

Eye opening: criteria for score

The assessment of eye opening shows that the arousal mechanisms located in the brainstem are functioning (Jennett and Teasdale, 1974). The best response is when the patient opens his/her eyes spontaneously and scores 4. If the patient opens his/her eyes in response to speech, the score is 3.

If a patient opens his/her eyes to painful stimuli, the score is 2. If there is no response, even to painful stimuli, the score is 1. Painful stimuli should be applied as a means of safeguarding the patient's wellbeing and can be applied in three ways:

⌘ *Trapezius pinch*. Take approximately 5 cm of the trapezius muscle between the thumb and the forefinger and twist
⌘ *Supraorbital pressure*. Feel the orbital rim and apply pressure to the orbital ridge to stimulate the supraorbital nerve (avoid if facial fractures suspected)
⌘ *Sternal rub*. Rub the centre of the sternum using the knuckles of a clenched fist.

Verbal response: criteria for score

The verbal response assesses consciousness by ascertaining whether the patient is aware of him/herself and the environment:

⌘ *Orientated*. For patients to be orientated, they must be able to tell the observer who they are, where they are, the day/date and why they are where they are (Jennett and Teasdale, 1974). A patient who is orientated scores 5
⌘ *Confused*. If the patient is able to converse but is not orientated the score is 4. The patient may be able to hold a conversation with the observer but cannot accurately answer all the questions
⌘ *Inappropriate speech*. If a patient only replies in monosyllables or phrases that make little or no sense, the patient will score 3
⌘ *Incomprehensible speech*. The patient is less aware of the environment, and his/her verbal responses may be in the form of incomprehensible sounds. If the patient responds only with sounds, the score is 2. Verbal and painful stimuli may be required
⌘ *No response*. If there is no verbal response to either verbal or painful stimulus, the score is 1.

Best motor response: criteria for score

⌘ *Following a command*. If patients can obey a command, the score is 6. If patients do not follow commands, further assessment involves the use of a painful stimulus to determine response
⌘ *Localizing to pain*. If the patient responds to a central painful stimulus and attempts to remove the source of the pain, the score is 5
⌘ *Flexes to pain*. When a central painful stimulus is applied, patients may flex/bend their arm towards the source of the pain but are not able to localize the pain or remove the source of the pain. Flexion to pain will give a score of 4
⌘ *Abnormal flexion*. In response to a central painful stimulus, the patient will bend his/her arm and rotate the wrist, resulting in a spastic posture. An abnormal flexion response scores 3
⌘ *Abnormal extension*. In response to a central painful stimulus, the patient will extend his/her arms or may rotate the arm inwards and will score 2
⌘ *No response*. The patient has no motor response to central pain and scores 1.

Assessment of pupillary response

Examination of the pupils and their reaction to light is a vital additional assessment, which indicates raised intracranial pressure (ICP) resulting in compression of the cranial nerves (oculomotor nerve). Assessment of the pupil can be carried out in both conscious and unconscious patients (*Box 8.4*).

Box 8.4: Guideline for recording pupil reaction

⌘ Inform and explain procedure to patient

⌘ Wash hands

⌘ Darken environment if possible

⌘ Hold both eyes open and note the shape and size of both pupils: normally pupils are round and the average size is 2–5 mm. Both pupils should be equal in size. If pupils are dilated, it is a sign of raised intracranial pressure. Close eyes in unconscious patient in order to prevent corneal damage

⌘ Holding one eye open, move a bright light from the outer aspect of the eye towards the pupil — the pupils should constrict. Remove the light source and the pupil should dilate to its original size

⌘ Repeat for the other eye

⌘ Record observation and report any changes.

Assessment of the pupil involves:

⌘ Looking at the shape of both pupils
⌘ Looking at the size of the pupils
⌘ Looking at the reaction to light.

Consensual light reflex

To assess consensual light reflex, hold both eyelids open and shine the light in the same way as above. The pupils in both eyes should constrict equally.

Vital signs

Vital signs form part of the neurological assessment (*Figure 8.2*); as the centres for the vital signs are located in the brainstem, damage to this area can affect their function:

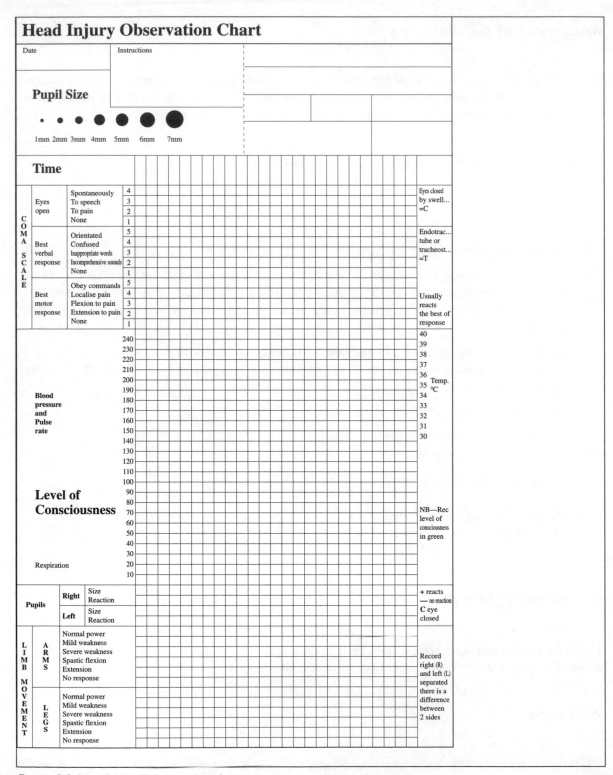

Figure 8.2: Head injury observation chart

⌘ *Blood pressure and pulse.* As the ICP rises, the brain becomes hypoxic and ischaemic. To counteract this effect and to perfuse the brain, the body responds by increasing the arterial blood pressure. This results in the patient becoming bradycardic

⌘ *Respiration.* If the brainstem is affected, there will be changes in the rate and pattern of breathing. Apnoea and Cheyne–Stokes breathing are caused by the sudden rise in ICP

⌘ *Temperature.* Damage to the hypothalamus may result in alterations in temperature control.

Limb movements

Both arms and legs should be assessed for normal power, mild weakness, severe weakness, spastic flexion, extension and no response. This may indicate damage to the brain and spinal cord.

Post-procedure

⌘ Document findings on a chart
⌘ Inform medical staff of any significant changes.

References

Bassett C (1997) Medical investigations 1: lumbar puncture. *Br J Nurs* **6:** 405–6

Blows W (2002) Diagnostic investigations. Part 1: lumbar puncture. *Nurs Times* **98**(36): 25–6

Hickey JV (1997) *The Clinical Practice of Neurological and Neurosurgical Nursing.* Lippincott Williams and Wilkins, Philadelphia

Jennett B, Teasdale G (1974) Assessment of coma and impaired consciousness. *Lancet* **2:** 81–4

Jennett B, Teasdale G (1981) *Management of Head Injuries: Contemporary Neurology Series.* Davies, Philadelphia

National Institute for Clinical Excellence (2003) *Head Injury, Triage, Assessment, Investigations and Early Management of Head Injury in Infants, Children and Adults: Clinical Guidelines 4.* NICE, London

Shah S (1999) Neurological assessment. *Nurs Stand* **13**(22): 49–56

Tate J, Tasota FJ (2000) Eye on diagnostics: looking at lumbar puncture in adults. *Nursing* **30**(11): 91

Further reading

Cree C (2003) Acquired brain injury: acute management. *Nurs Stand* **18**(11): 45–54

Woodrow P (2000) Head injuries: acute care. *Nurs Stand* **14**(35): 37–44

Chapter 9

Renal system

Continuous ambulatory peritoneal dialysis

Peritoneal dialysis is a procedure whereby a physiological solution (dialysate) is infused into the peritoneal cavity. The peritoneum acts as a semi-permeable membrane through which dialysis occurs. During dialysis, molecules move from the bloodstream, across the peritoneum and into the dialysate (and *vice versa*) by a process known as diffusion. Osmosis also occurs across the peritoneum, resulting in the removal of excess water.

Peritoneal dialysis occurs constantly within the patient. The patient must change the fluid every 4–6 hours throughout the day, every day of the week. This is known as performing an 'exchange'. If the exchanges of used dialysate for fresh dialysate are not performed, equilibrium will occur within the dwelling dialysate and diffusion of toxins will not occur.

In order to enable peritoneal dialysis to occur, access to the peritoneal cavity has to be gained. A minor operation is performed, either under local or general anaesthetic, and a soft, plastic Tenckhoff catheter is inserted into the abdomen. The tube is called the peritoneal dialysis (PD) catheter and is permanent.

The catheter is held in place by the body's own production of fibrous tissue. The catheter has two fabric cuffs known as Dacron cuffs. One of the cuffs is placed just beneath the skin and the other is placed deep inside the abdomen, just outside the peritoneal cavity (Stein and Wild, 2002). Fibrous tissue develops on the cuffs and provides a strong anchor for the catheter. The fibrous tissue also seals the peritoneal cavity, thus protecting it from infection and preventing dialysate from leaking out. About 15 cm of the catheter remains outside the patient and provides the means for attaching the bags of dialysis fluid.

PD catheters may be used immediately if necessary; however, a 10–14 day waiting period is generally practised to promote healing, thus preventing leakage of dialysate (Zabat, 2003).

Reasons for the procedure

⌘ Removes waste products from blood for those patients in renal failure
⌘ Prevents complications caused by toxicity
⌘ As an alternative to haemodialysis.

Pre-procedure

Equipment required

- ⌘ Alcohol wipes and hand gel
- ⌘ Gloves
- ⌘ Warm dialysate bag (to 37°C) of correct type and strength according to the prescription
- ⌘ Bucket
- ⌘ PD-giving set
- ⌘ Drip stand
- ⌘ Clamps
- ⌘ Sterile cover
- ⌘ Water thermometer
- ⌘ Towels.

Specific patient preparation required

- ⌘ Assess for abdominal pain and pyrexia as these may indicate infection (peritonitis)
- ⌘ Observe PD catheter site for signs of infection (redness, discharge)
- ⌘ Do not proceed with the exchange if the patient has signs and symptoms of peritonitis or infection at the exit site, and contact medical staff
- ⌘ The patient may either lie down or be seated for the procedure.

During the procedure

Setting up the PD set

- ⌘ The packaging on all equipment should be checked and be intact
- ⌘ Place bucket on floor
- ⌘ Thoroughly wash and dry hands
- ⌘ Open the outer cover of the dialysate bag and expose the outlet port
- ⌘ Suspend dialysate bag on drip stand
- ⌘ Attach the giving set to the dialysate bag
- ⌘ Turn the flow rate on to prime the giving set. Once completed turn the flow rate off
- ⌘ Apply alcohol handrub to hands and put on gloves
- ⌘ Pull protective cover from the end of the tubing. Take care not to contaminate the exposed end
- ⌘ Remove the sterile cover from the end of the PD catheter
- ⌘ Attach the dialysate bag tubing to the PD catheter, using the Luer–Lok mechanism (*Figure 9.1*).

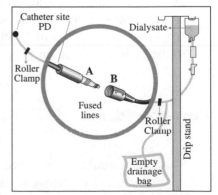

Figure 9.1: Attach dialysate bag to catheter

Procedure for draining dialysate out

⌘ Put a clamp onto each of the dialysate lines and break the seal inside the dialysis fluid lines

⌘ Hang the full bag of unused dialysate on the drip stand and place the empty drainage bag into the bucket

⌘ Open the twist clamp on the PD catheter and undo the clamp attached to the line entering the drainage bag

⌘ Used dialysate should flow from the patient into the drainage bag. The patient should be asked whether he/she is experiencing any pain or discomfort on draining out. If the patient experiences problems draining out, a change in his/her position may encourage a movement of the catheter within the abdominal cavity and thereby improve drainage. Fibrin clots may also impede the flow from the catheter and may require heparinization of the dialysate

⌘ The used dialysate should be observed for cloudiness, which may indicate peritonitis. If this occurs, medical advice must be sought before commencing the 'fill' procedure. The cloudy bag must be sent to the laboratory for analysis

⌘ Document the time of drainage commencement

⌘ When the drainage tube feels cold to the touch and the drainage bag is full of fluid, drainage is complete

⌘ Once drainage is complete, the twist clamp on the PD catheter should be closed.

Procedure for draining dialysate in

⌘ The clamp on the line leading from the unused dialysate bag on the drip stand should be opened for approximately 15 seconds to allow fresh dialysate to run into the drainage bag. This will prevent re-circulation of used dialysate

⌘ A clamp should then be applied to the line leading to the drainage bag, thereby closing it off

⌘ The twist clamp on the PD catheter should be opened, allowing fresh dialysate to fill the peritoneal cavity

⌘ Document time of commencement of fill

⌘ Once filling is complete, the twist clamp should be closed

⌘ Open the sterile cover packet and apply alcohol handrub to hands and wait to dry

⌘ Disconnect the PD catheter from the dialysate bags, keeping the PD catheter in the hand to avoid contamination. Drop the dialysate line into the bucket

⌘ Apply the sterile cover to the PD catheter securely. The PD catheter should then be securely taped to the patient's abdomen to prevent trauma.

Post-procedure

⌘ The bag containing the used dialysate should be weighed and the result recorded on the appropriate chart. The weight should be compared with that of the original infusion. If the used dialysate weighs more than the initial dialysate weight, ultrafiltration of excess fluid has occurred. A lower weight of the used dialysate compared with the original infusion may indicate either that some fluid has been retained within the patient because of drainage problems, or that the fluid has been absorbed by the patient

⌘ If the used dialysate is not contaminated, it should be disposed of in the same manner as other bodily fluids

⌘ Daily weight

⌘ Time of commencement and completion of each exchange

⌘ Time of start and finish of drainage time

⌘ Accurate fluid balance after each complete exchange

⌘ Observe the nature of the fluid drained, i.e. fibrin, cloudy, clear

⌘ Monitor for complications.

Obtaining a catheter specimen of urine

A catheter specimen of urine (CSU) is the collection of a clean, uncontaminated sample of urine via an indwelling urethral catheter. This can be investigated by the microbiology department to identify any pathological changes and subsequently inform treatment. The specimen of urine needs to be taken from urine present in the bladder. Urine that has collected in the catheter bag may have been contaminated with bacteria, e.g. bacteria could have been introduced into the catheter bag when it had been emptied (Ward, 1997). This can give a false–positive result and subsequent inappropriate treatment.

Reasons for the procedure

⌘ To determine the presence of urinary tract infection

⌘ To identify suitable antibiotic therapy.

Pre-procedure

Equipment required

⌘ 20 ml syringe

⌘ Alcohol wipe

⌘ 21-gauge syringe needle

⌘ Catheter clamp

⌘ Pre-labelled sterile container

⌘ Clean gloves

⌘ Apron

⌘ Microbiology request form

⌘ Sharps disposal box
⌘ Spare catheter drainage bag, if required
⌘ Tray.

Specific patient preparation required

⌘ The patient does not need to be moved into a particular position; the nurse needs access to the catheter drainage bag port, ensuring the patient's dignity and privacy at all times
⌘ The urethral catheter is continually draining urine into the bag. To allow the fluid volume to build up in the bladder, the catheter needs to be temporarily clamped. The clamp should be positioned next to the port (the clamp should not be applied directly to the urinary catheter). Poole (2002) identified that 1 ml urine is adequate for microbiological purposes.

During the procedure

⌘ Put on protective clothing
⌘ Assemble the syringe and needle
⌘ Clean the catheter port with an alcohol wipe and allow to dry
⌘ Unsheathe and insert the needle into the sample port at a 90° angle. Stop pushing the needle once the bevel can be seen inside the lumen and urine can be aspirated
⌘ Withdraw the plunger and aspirate the required sample
⌘ Remove the needle from the sample port and dispose it in the sharps bin
⌘ Open the sterile container, press down on the plunger of the syringe and squeeze the collected urine into the container
⌘ Close the container and dispose of the syringe
⌘ Unclamp the catheter bag tubing. Inspect for damage and replace bag as necessary.

Post-procedure

⌘ Remove protective clothing
⌘ Date and time specimen container and request form
⌘ Place container and request form in the appropriate microbiology bag and transfer to laboratory according to local policy
⌘ Document collection of the specimen in the patient notes.

Student skill laboratory activity

⌘ Assemble equipment required for CSU
⌘ Practise the skill of inserting a needle into a catheter port
⌘ Withdraw a mock sample and transfer into a sterile container
⌘ Discuss when other types of containers may be used for a CSU.

Obtaining a midstream specimen of urine

A midstream specimen of urine (MSU) is often taken following detection of abnormalities from the urinalysis. A midstream specimen may also be collected if the patient is known to have an existing urinary tract infection. The sample is sent to the laboratory for microscopy, culture and sensitivity testing:

⌘ It is first examined under the microscope for abnormalities, such as blood cells and white cells
⌘ Culture refers to the incubation of the sample, to encourage organism growth. This will determine whether there is a specific infective agent causing the abnormality
⌘ Sensitivity is when the cultured growth is tested with various treatment agents, such as specific antibiotics, to determine which one is most effective for eliminating the organism
⌘ The results are reported to the medical team, to enable them to prescribe the most appropriate treatment.

Reasons for the procedure

⌘ The aim is to catch the middle part of the urine flow from a single void. During this process the specimen is less likely to be contaminated as the urethral area will have been flushed through from the initial stream of urine (Baillie and Arrowsmith, 2001).

Pre-procedure

Equipment required

⌘ Sterile container for collection of the urine sample, clearly labelled with the name of the patient and date of collection
⌘ Disposable gloves
⌘ Apron
⌘ Sterile specimen pot appropriate for the investigations being undertaken
⌘ Cleansing agents as required
⌘ Laboratory request form.

Specific patient preparation required

⌘ Provision of a suitable private environment (toilet facilities/bathroom) with handwashing facilities for the patient to produce the urine specimen without interruptions (Cook, 1996)
⌘ Encourage the patient to wash his/her hands before and after voiding to reduce the incidence of sample contamination
⌘ Instruct or assist the patient to cleanse the genital and urethral meatus area.

During the procedure

⌘ Void the initial stream of urine (approximately 30–60 ml) into the toilet/commode, then stop and collect the middle part of the stream of urine (20 ml) into the container. The patient should then complete urinating in the toilet/commode (Elley and Semple, 1999).

Post-procedure

⌘ Label the sample container with the patient's details — name, identity number, address, date of birth and time collected
⌘ Remove gloves and apron and wash hands thoroughly
⌘ Complete the appropriate laboratory form with the details as required
⌘ Place the sample container in a plastic specimen bag with the completed form and ensure that it is transported promptly to the laboratory
⌘ Place sample in specimen refrigerator
⌘ Inform the patient that the sample has been obtained successfully and that the outcome of the test will be relayed to them in due course
⌘ Document the collection of the specimen in the patient's nursing records.

Student skill laboratory activity

⌘ Identify the equipment that you would require to collect a midstream specimen of urine
⌘ Discuss some of the difficulties that patients may experience with this procedure.

Female urethral catheterization

Female catheterization involves a urethral catheter being placed into the bladder using an aseptic technique. It is secured in place for a period of time with an inflated balloon at the distal tip of the catheter.

Reasons for the procedure

Female patients may require an indwelling urethral catheter for a variety of reasons, including urine retention, pre- and postoperative management and accurate urine measurement or urodynamic investigations (Robinson, 2001). Eustice (2004) identified postpartum urinary retention as a common rationale for short-term female urethral catheterization.

Pre-procedure

Equipment required

⌘   Select appropriate catheter (*Table 9.1*)

Table 9.1: Catheter selection

Type	Duration	Available catheter material	Range of lengths	Diameter size
Short-term	Up to 2 weeks	Plastic latex	23–26 cm 30 cm	Selection dependent on the purpose of catheterization, e.g. smallest diameter catheter to drain urine, and larger size catheter when haematuria is present
Medium-term	Up to 4 weeks	Polytetrafluroethylene	40–44 cm	
Long-term	Up to 12 weeks	Hydrogel Silicone Silver-coated		

From Lowthian (1998); Pomfret (2000)

⌘   Clean working surface/trolley
⌘   Catheter pack
⌘   Urinary catheter of the appropriate size and material
⌘   Cleansing agent, such as sterile water
⌘   Sterile lubricant and/or single-use anaesthetic gel, as these can reduce trauma caused by catheterization and improve patient comfort (Pellowe, 2001)
⌘   Catheter drainage bag
⌘   Catheter stand that secures the catheter bag off the floor
⌘   Fluid balance chart.

Specific patient preparation required

⌘   The woman should be positioned in as comfortable a position as possible as she may be in that position for several minutes, thus ascertaining any joint or back problems for the patient is important. The usual position for the women is the dorsal recumbent position with knees bent and supported and her feet approximately 60 cm apart. Alternatively, the patient can lay on her side with her legs bent towards her chest; the visualization of the genitalia would be from behind. This would be more beneficial for the elderly, who may have lower lumbar problems

✿ Doherty (2000) advocates cleansing the genital area before catheterization, although Bennett (2002) suggests that washing the genitals with mild soap and water is adequate. The general consensus is that the genital area should be socially clean; further measures should be applied if the women is menstruating or has heavy vaginal discharge. Genitalia should be cleansed around the labia majora, labia minora and the urethral opening from an anterior to posterior direction, therefore minimizing bacterial contamination to the urethral meatus.

During the procedure

✿ A sterile field is established by opening the catheter pack on a previously cleaned area, usually a metal trolley. The nurse places the necessary equipment on the sterile field without touching and contaminating the area. With all of the equipment prepared, the nurse puts on the correct-sized sterile gloves before coming into contact with the patient

✿ A local anaesthetic gel in a pre-filled syringe can be introduced into the female urethra to reduce discomfort and act as a lubricant, so reducing the surface friction between the catheter surface and the urethral wall (Doherty, 1999). It is also an opportunity to identify and visualize the urethral meatus before catheter insertion (*Figure 9.2*)

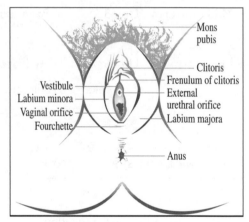

Figure 9.2: Urethral meatus

✿ The catheter is slowly inserted into the urethra and into the bladder. To promote relaxation of the urinary sphincter and reduce discomfort, encourage the patient to take deep breaths in and out. Once the catheter is inserted successfully into the bladder, urine will flow from the external tubing; a receiver should be positioned to collect it for measurement and possible testing with a urinalysis stick

✿ Inflation of the balloon with sterile water secures it to the bladder. The balloon infill can vary from 2.5 ml for a paediatric catheter to 30 ml for a standard female catheter. Overinflation of the balloon can cause damage to the bladder trigone. Generally 5–10 ml adequately secures the balloon into the bladder

✿ Connect catheter to drainage system and secure appropriately.

Post-procedure

✿ Record in the patient's documentation details of the urinary catheter inserted. The batch number and expiry date of the catheter needs to be documented

⌘ Inform the patient that she can move with the catheter in place (as long as this is within her capabilities), and that walking around will not dislodge or impede the flow of urine. Discuss how the patient feels after the insertion of the catheter, whether she has any discomfort or pain. This may indicate urethral trauma

⌘ Observe the flow of urine into the catheter bag; observe the colour, smell of urine and any indications of infection. If necessary, take a catheter specimen of urine and send to microbiology

⌘ Maintain an accurate fluid balance chart and report significant changes

⌘ When the catheter bag is emptied, clean gloves should be worn and the urine accurately measured, documented and disposed of appropriately.

Removal of the urinary catheter

⌘ The indwelling urethral catheter should be removed at night, preferably between 10:00pm and midnight (Fernandez et al, 2003). This results in the patient voiding normally, with a smaller chance of urinary retention

⌘ The balloon should be completely deflated by using a syringe and aspirating the fluid at the inflation port

⌘ The catheter should then be removed slowly and gently to prevent trauma

⌘ After removal of the catheter, document its removal in the patient's documentation noting any significant observations of the catheter

⌘ Inform the patient where the nearest toilet is situated and provide a receptacle to be placed in the toilet so the urine can be measured and documented

⌘ Monitor when the patient first passes urine.

Student skill laboratory activity

⌘ Assemble the equipment you would require for female urinary catheterization

⌘ Select an appropriate simulation manikin and practise the skill of female urinary catheterization

⌘ Practise removing the catheter

⌘ Discuss some of the issues that should be considered throughout the procedure and in relation to transcultural nursing.

Male catheterization

Urinary catheterization is the insertion of a tube into the bladder via the urethra and is performed using an aseptic technique (Wilson and Waugh, 2001; Marieb, 2004). It may also be taught to the patient, using a clean procedure, as intermittent self-catheterization.

Reasons for the procedure

⌘ Relieve acute retention of urine
⌘ After incomplete bladder emptying
⌘ Measurement of residual if bladder scanning is unavailable
⌘ Bypass obstruction
⌘ Instillation of catheter maintenance solutions or medications
⌘ Enable bladder function tests (urodynamics) to be performed
⌘ Allow irrigation of the bladder
⌘ Pre- and postoperative bladder drainage
⌘ Accurate urine measurement in the severely ill
⌘ Management of incontinence in the terminally ill, in last stages of life
⌘ Intractable incontinence where other methods are unsuitable or have failed.

Pre-procedure

Equipment required

⌘ Clean working surface/trolley
⌘ Sterile pack suitable for catheterization (containing gallipot, tray, gauze swabs, paper towels, sterile field)
⌘ Syringes, needles and 10 ml sterile water suitable for injection if not using catheter with pre-filled balloon
⌘ Analgesic antiseptic lubricant gel containing 11 ml lidocaine hydrochloride 2% (Ogden, 2003)
⌘ Normal saline or mild antiseptic for cleansing meatus
⌘ Sterile gloves (two pairs)
⌘ Sterile standard length (40–44 cm) urinary catheter of the appropriate material (*Box 9.1*)

Box 9.1: Choice of catheter

Size Catheter size is determined in both length and diameter of lumen depending on the nature of the problem for which it is being introduced

Length Standard (male) length (40–44 cm), unless the length of the penis determines the shorter (female) length (23–26 cm). Determine the length of catheter, which may extrude from the meatus, and consider which may be easier for the patient to accommodate in clothing without kinking and be less obtrusive (Robinson, 2001)

Diameter Size 12–16 Ch unless the procedure is for instillation or drainage of fluids other than urine or following prostatectomy when up to size 18 Ch may be necessary. The smallest size that provides adequate drainage should be chosen

Box 9.1 continued on next page

Box 9.1 *continued*: Choice of catheter

Type	For short-term use (up to 4 weeks), polytetrafluoroethylene (PTFE) coated may be appropriate; for long-term use (up to 3 months), hydrogel-coated, silicone elastomer-coated latex or 100% silicone should be used. All-silicone should always be used if the patient has a latex allergy (Woodward, 1997)
Balloon type	Catheters may have integral pre-filled balloon for ease of use. For non-prefilled catheters, 10 ml infill is generally used, but 30 ml may be used to aid postoperative haemostasis by applying pressure to the bladder neck. Leakage of urine from around the bladder neck has been associated with balloon volumes over 10 ml (Winn, 1996)

Check expiry date and for signs of deterioration caused by storage

---

⌘ Catheter valve, catheter drainage bag, support accessories (*Box 9.2*)
⌘ Clamp.

Box 9.2: Factors affecting choice of valve or bag use and types of support accessories

The patient may have increased quality of life if given the choice of a valve (Woods et al, 1999). If there are no potential medical complications, offer the patient a valve if he has satisfactory:

⌘ Bladder sensation
⌘ Capacity of bladder
⌘ Cognitive function
⌘ Dexterity

Selection of drainage bag is determined by:

⌘ Capacity required
⌘ Fixation position
⌘ Length of inlet tubing
⌘ Potential weight of full bag
⌘ Ability of patient to manage valve emptying
⌘ Patient choice
⌘ Frequency of monitoring urinary output

Types of support accessories:

⌘ Leg straps
⌘ Leg sleeve
⌘ Sporan
⌘ Catheter stand
⌘ Catheter bed holder

Specific patient preparation required

⌘ The procedure will be facilitated if the patient has a full bladder
⌘ Assist the patient into the supine position with the legs extended
⌘ Place protective sheet under the patient's buttocks and adjust lighting as necessary
⌘ If necessary, using universal precautions assist patient to wash genitalia with soap and water, paying particular attention to the glans and meatus to remove accumulated smegma. Dry well.

During the procedure

⌘ Open sterile pack and put on sterile gloves
⌘ If not using pre-filled balloon, draw up 10 ml sterile water into syringe and dispose of needle safely
⌘ Apply the sterile drapes appropriately
⌘ With your non-dominant hand lift the penis (this hand is now considered contaminated and should maintain a firm grasp until the procedure is completed). Hold the penis gently and laterally behind the glans with a sterile swab
⌘ Anaesthetize the urethra with 11 ml local anaesthetic gel, instilling slowly. Allow 5 minutes to elapse for the gel to take effect, keeping the urethral meatus closed with gentle digital pressure to prevent leakage and facilitate complete urethral lubrication
⌘ Place a sterile tray inbetween the patient's legs to receive the urine drainage
⌘ Open the inner cover of the catheter, but do not remove the catheter
⌘ Using a gauze swab, hold the penis with slight upward tension and at a 90° angle from the pelvis to reduce the acute angle of the bulbar urethra. Using the inner cover of the catheter to maintain sterility, gently insert the catheter until urine starts to flow into the tray
⌘ If resistance is felt at the prostate, ask the patient to cough to assist the passage of the catheter through the prostatic urethra
⌘ Check for urine drainage
⌘ Insert the catheter a further 1–2 cm to avoid balloon inflation in the urethra and inflate the balloon with sterile water. Underinflated balloons may occlude the drainage holes of the catheter or cause distortion of the catheter tip, leading to irritation and trauma to the bladder wall (Pomfret, 1999)
⌘ Observe for signs of pain, discomfort and urethral bleeding
⌘ Once the balloon is inflated, gently withdraw the catheter until slight resistance is felt
⌘ Attach a sterile, closed drainage system or valve. Gravity is important for drainage and the prevention of urine backflow. Ensure that catheter bags are always draining downwards, do not become kinked and are secured and below bladder level
⌘ Ensure the foreskin (if present) is replaced back over the glans
⌘ Make the patient comfortable and ensure area is dry
⌘ Stop and seek further advice if any of the following occur:
  – the catheter, during any stage of insertion, cannot be easily passed
  – the patient complains of undue pain
  – bleeding other than that normally associated with minor trauma.

Post–procedure

⌘ Dispose of equipment and dispose of any urine drained as per clinical waste policy and wash hands

⌘ Monitor urine output. Rapid drainage of large volumes of urine from the bladder may result in hypotension and/or haemorrhage (Upson, 1995). Clamp catheter if the volume drained is 1000 ml or greater. After 20 minutes release the clamp and allow urine to drain. If the amount of urine is 1000 ml or greater, repeat the clamping procedure

⌘ Document procedure (*Box 9.3*) and report any urethral trauma

---

Box 9.3: Information to be documented

Reason for catheterization

Type of catheterization

Type of catheter/manufacturer/batch number/expiry date

Catheter material/length/size/balloon size

Anaesthetic gel used

Drainage system used

Date and time of insertion

Date of planned catheter change

Evaluation date/review of care

Advice to patient/carer

Any complications

Interventions, where appropriate

⌘ Ongoing monitoring of possible complications such as urinary tract infection, encrustation, kinking of tubing, overflow and paraphimosis

⌘ Give advice and education to patient on the care of the catheter to prevent complications (Evans, 1999) and address issues in relation to lifestyle.

Student skill laboratory activity

⌘ Assemble the equipment you would require to undertake male catherization

⌘ Practise male catheterization on a manikin.

Urinalysis

Urinalysis is the testing of freshly voided urine for abnormalities. The collection, examination and testing of urine samples using reagent strips is a simple and reliable method for the diagnosis and screening of several conditions. Urine testing can be carried out in a variety of different settings, such as hospitals, GP surgeries or in the patient's home, as minimal equipment is needed. It is a relatively cheap screening tool, which can provide vital information on a number of different body systems. The precision of the reagent strips relies on the nurse accurately timing and reading the 'colour reaction change' that takes place once the strips have been dipped into the urine sample (Cook, 1996).

Reasons for the procedure

⌘ For diagnostic purposes (*Box 9.4*)
⌘ To monitor the effectiveness of treatment
⌘ To establish a baseline.

Box 9.4: Substances screened for during routine urinalysis

Substance	Terminology	Indication
Blood	Haematuria	Urinary tract infection, bladder/prostate cancer, menstruation
Glucose	Glycosuria	Diabetes mellitus or diseases reducing renal absorption, such as Cushing's syndrome, stress or acute pancreatitis
Ketones	Ketonuria	Diabetes mellitus or anorexia as it indicates the breakdown of fatty acids
Leucocytes		Urinary tract infection
Nitrites		Urinary tract infection
Protein (albumin, globulin)	Proteinuria	Urinary tract infection, hypertension, congestive cardiac failure, renal disease, diabetes
Specific gravity		A low specific gravity (below 1002) could indicate diabetes insipidus and anti-diuretic hormone resistance
Urobilinogen		Liver disease, bile duct obstruction, excessive destruction of red blood cells

---

Pre–procedure

Equipment required

- ✼ Clean container for collection of the urine sample, clearly labelled with the name of the patient and the date of collection
- ✼ Gloves to protect the nurse from possible infection and to adhere to standard precautions
- ✼ Watch with a second hand for accuracy of timing analyte reaction
- ✼ Reagent strips stored in the appropriate airtight manufacturer's container. Take the container holding the reagent testing strips and check to see that the use-by date has not expired
- ✼ Paper and pen (kept solely in the sluice area) to record test results immediately
- ✼ Recording chart to document the findings.

Specific patient preparation required

- ✼ Provision of a suitable private environment (toilet facilities/bathroom) with handwashing facilities for the patient to produce the urine specimen without interruptions (Cook, 1996)
- ✼ Encourage the patient to wash his/her hands before and after voiding to reduce the incidence of sample contamination.

During the procedure

- ✼ Take the sample to the appropriate area for testing, so that the equipment is to hand and the sample can be disposed of appropriately after it has been tested
- ✼ Observe the colour of the urine before testing. It should be yellow, straw coloured and clear in appearance; cloudiness or 'turbidity' may indicate the presence of abnormal cells and the likelihood of infection (Cook, 1996)
- ✼ Note the odour of the sample before testing. It should be odourless if it is a freshly voided sample
- ✼ Remove a single reagent-testing strip from the container and firmly replace the lid after this. Most strips must be stored in cool, dry, airtight conditions to ensure accuracy of results obtained
- ✼ To use the reagent strip, consult and follow the specific manufacturer's instructions as each may vary slightly. Note in particular the specified time required to read the individual reagent pads
- ✼ Avoid handling the test pads as this can influence the findings
- ✼ The reagent strip is dipped into the specimen of urine, ensuring that all reagent pads are covered. Remove the strip immediately from the urine
- ✼ Either gently tap the strip against the edge of the sample container or run the edge of the strip against the rim of the container to remove any excess urine. The strip should be held horizontally at this point to prevent urine running from test pad to test pad
- ✼ Timing starts when the strip is removed from the urine and the time intervals specified for each of the test pads scrupulously observed using the watch

⌘ The reagent strip can be read by holding it vertically or horizontally against the comparison chart produced on the container. After testing, the urine should be disposed of in the sluice or toilet

⌘ The sample container and reagent strip should be disposed of in a yellow plastic clinical waste bag

⌘ The nurse should record the result instantly

⌘ Finally the nurse should remove gloves and wash hands thoroughly.

Post-procedure

⌘ Record the results in the patient documentation

⌘ Report any abnormalities so that irregularities can be acted on promptly

⌘ Inform the patient of the findings

⌘ Note drugs being taken by the patient that could affect the result (*Box 9.5*).

Box 9.5: Factors that may influence the results

Factor	Alteration in
Excessive amounts of certain food substances, e.g. beetroot	Colour — urine may be pink/red
Fluid intake	Specific gravity — low if fluid intake is high
	Colour — becomes darker the lower the amount of fluid consumed
Altitude	Specific gravity — becomes lower, the higher the altitude
Environmental temperature/humidity	Specific gravity — becomes higher, the higher the temperature
Phenothiazides, e.g. chlorpromazine	Bilirubin — false–positive
Phenolphthalein bromsulphthalein, e.g. L-dopa metabolites	Ketones — false–positive
Container contaminated with bleach	Blood — false–positive
Skin preparation with povidine iodine	Blood — false–positive

Student skill laboratory activity

⌘ Practise urine testing in the laboratory using artificially prepared solutions

⌘ Collect data from six other colleagues and discuss the reliability and accuracy of the tests.

References

Baillie L, Arrowsmith V (2001) Meeting elimination needs. In: Baillie L, ed. *Developing Practical Nursing Skills*. Arnold, London

Bennett C (2002) Comparison of bladder management complication outcomes in female spinal cord injury patients. *J Urol* **153**: 1458–60

Cook R (1996) Urinalysis: ensuring accurate urine testing. *Nurs Stand* **10**(46): 49–52

Doherty W (1999) Instillagel: an anaesthetic gel for use in catheterisation. *Br J Nurs* **8**: 109–12

Doherty W (2000) Intermittent catheterisation: draining the bladder. *Nurs Times Plus* **96**(31): 13

Elley K, Semple M (1999) Collecting a mid-stream specimen of urine. *Nurs Times* **95**(2): suppl 1–2

Eustice S (2004) Management of voiding difficulties associated with pregnancy. *Nurs Times* **100**(12): 50–2

Evans E (1999) Indwelling catheter care: dispelling the misconceptions. *Geriatr Nurs* **20**(2): 85–8

Fernandez R, Griffiths R, Murie P (2003) Comparison of late night and early morning removal of short-term catheters. *JBI Reports* **1**: 1–16

Lowthian P (1998) The dangers of long-term catheter drainage. *Br J Nurs* **4**: 328–34

Marieb EN (2004) *Human Anatomy and Physiology*. 6th edn. Pearson Benjamin Cummings, San Francisco

Ogden V (2003) Anaesthetic gel insertion during male catheterisation. *J Community Nurs* **17**(1): 4–8

Pellowe C (2001) Preventing infections from short-term indwelling catheters. *Nurs Times* **97**(14): 34–5

Pomfret I (1999) Catheter care. *Primary Health Care* **9**(5): 29–36

Pomfret I (2000) Catheter care in the community. *Nurs Stand* **14**(27): 46–51

Poole C (2002) Diagnosis and management of urinary tract infection in children. *Nurs Stand* **16**(38): 47–52

Robinson J (2001) Urethral catheter selection. *Nurs Stand* **15**(25): 39–42

Stein A, Wild J (2002) *Kidney Dialysis and Transplants*. Class Publishing, London

Upson C (1995) Catheter clamping after catheterisation and rapid urine loss. *Urol Nurs* **15**: 63–4

Ward V (1997) *Preventing Hospital-acquired Infection: Clinical Guidelines*. Public Health Laboratory Service, London

Wilson KJW, Waugh A (2001) *Ross and Wilson: Anatomy and Physiology in Health and Illness*. 9th edn. Churchill Livingstone, Edinburgh

Winn C (1996) Basing catheter care on research principles. *Nurs Stand* **10**(18): 38–40

Woods M, McCreanor J, Aitchison M (1999) An assessment of urethral catheter valves. *Prof Nurse* **14**: 72–4

Woodward S (1997) Complications of allergies to latex urinary catheters. *Br J Nurs* **6**: 786–93

Zabat E (2003) When your patient needs peritoneal dialysis. *Nursing* **33**(8): 52–4

Further reading

Baxter Healthcare Corporation (2001) *Physioneal CAPD Exchange Procedure Guide*. Baxter, Newbury

Buckley R (1999) Keep it legal. *Nurs Times* **95**(6): 75–9

Docherty B (2001) Clinical practice review. Urine collection and analysis. *Prof Nurse* **16**: 1076

Getliffe KA (1993) Care of urinary catheters. *Nurs Stand* **7**(44): 31–4

Getliffe K (1996) Care of urinary catheters. *Nurs Stand* **11**(11): 47–50

Govan ADT, McKay Hart D, Callander R (1993) *Gynaecology Illustrated*. 4th edn. Churchill Livingstone, London

Hayes D (2003) Performing peritoneal dialysis. *Nursing* **33**(3): 17

Howell AB (1998) Inhibition of the adherence of P-fimbriated *Escherichia coli* to uroepithelial cell surfaces by proanthocyanidin extracts from cranberries. *New Engl J Med* **339**: 1085–6

Kohler-Ockmore J, Feneley RNC (1990) *Long-term Urinary Catheterisation in the Community*. Bristol Health Authority, Bristol

Kunin CM (1989) Blockage of urinary catheters: role of microorganisms and constituents of the urine on formation of encrustation. *J Clin Epidemiol* **42**: 835–42

Lavender R (2000) Cranberry juice: the facts. *NT Plus* **96**(40): 11–12

Marieb EN (2003) *Essentials of Human Anatomy and Physiology*. Pearson Educational, New Jersey

National Institute of Clinical Excellence (2003) *Infection Control: Prevention of Healthcare Associated Infection in Primary and Community Care (Clinical Guideline 2)*. NICE, London

Nursing and Midwifery Council (1998) *Guidelines for Records and Record Keeping*. NMC, London

Pellowe C, Pratt R (2004) Catheter-associated urinary tract infections: primary care guidelines. *Nurs Times* **100**(2): 53–5

Pomfret IJ (1996) Catheters: design, selection and management. *Br J Nurs* **5**: 245–51

RCN Continence Care Forum (1997) *Male Catheterisation: The Role of the Nurse, Professional Accountability for Practice*. RCN, London

Robinson J (2001) Choosing a catheter. *J Community Nurs* **17**(3): 37–42

Roe B (1993) Catheter associated urinary tract infections: a review. *J Clin Nurs* **2**: 197–203

Roe B, Brocklehurst JC (1987) Study of patients with indwelling catheters. *J Adv Nurs* **12**: 713–18

Saint S, Lipsky BA (1999) Preventing catheter-related bacteriuria. Should we? Can we? *Arch Intern Med* **159**(8): 800–8

Shallcross P (2000) Male catheterisation and the extended role of the female nurse. *Br J Community Nurs* **5**(2): 81–5

Simpson L (2001) Indwelling urethral catheters. *Nurs Stand* **15**(46): 47–53

Simpson L (2001) Indwelling urethral catheters: reducing the risk of potential complications through proactive management. *Primary Health Care* **11**(2): 57–64

Stickler D (1993) Blockage of urethral catheters by bacterial biofilms. *J Infect* **27**: 133–5

Torrance C, Elley K (1998a) Urine testing, part 1: observation. Practical procedures for nurses supplement part 7.1. *Nurs Times* **94**(4)

Torrance C, Elley K (1998b) Urine testing, part 2: urinalysis. Practical procedures for nurses supplement part 7.2. *Nurs Times* **94**(5)

Warren JW (2001) Catheter associated urinary tract infections. *Int J Antimicrob Agents* **17**: 299–303

Wilde MH, Carrigan MJ (2003) A chart audit of factors related to urine flow and urinary tract infection. *J Adv Nurs* **43**: 254–62

Wilson J (1995) *Infection Control in Clinical Practice: In Preventing Infection Associated with Urethral Catheters*. Balliere Tindall, London

Winn C (1998) Complications with urinary catheters. *Prof Nurse* **13**(Suppl 5): S7–S10

Chapter 10

Miscellaneous

Aseptic technique

Aseptic technique or non-touch technique involves using sterile equipment, lotions and dressings to carry out clinical procedures such as catheterization, tracheal suctioning and wound dressing. All sterile equipment should be checked for integrity, evidence of sterility and expiry date. While the principles of asepsis will apply to most clinical procedures, in this section the aseptic technique described is that used to carry out a wound dressing.

Reasons for the procedure

⌘ To prevent the spread of infection by direct or indirect means (Xavier, 1999). The spread of infection includes the hands of clinical staff, inanimate objects (e.g. instruments and clothes) and dust particles or droplet micro-organisms. The nurse should therefore be mindful of these factors when carrying out the procedure
⌘ To prevent the introduction of micro-organisms
⌘ To promote healing.

Pre-procedure

Equipment required

⌘ Dressing trolley
⌘ Dressing pack, which may include items such as dressing drape, gauze swabs, gallipots, sterile gloves/disposable forceps and disposal bag (Sterile gloves are now largely used for dressings; however, for certain procedures such as removal of sutures, sterile forceps can be useful.)
⌘ Sterile disposable gloves (if not included in pack)
⌘ Alcohol handrub
⌘ Hypoallergenic tape
⌘ Additional dressings and wound-care products as required
⌘ Clean, disposable apron

⌘ Wash and dry own scissors and clean with alcohol swab (it is imperative that the scissors are not placed on the sterile field) if using these for cutting tape (Nicol et al, 2000)

⌘ Use sterile scissors if cutting dressings to fit

⌘ If using a 'sharp' such as a stitch cutter, a sharps bin should be placed on the bottom shelf of the trolley.

If cleansing or irrigation of the wound is required with normal saline

⌘ Warm cleansing/irrigation solution to body temperature (Jamieson et al, 2002) as it takes cells 40 minutes to recover from the use of cold fluid and for cell division to recommence (Myers, 1982). For this reason also, wounds should not be exposed for any longer than is necessary

⌘ Receiver to collect irrigation fluid

⌘ Cleansing/irrigation fluid. It is the general consensus that isotonic 0.9% saline is the fluid of choice for general wound cleansing or irrigation (Collier, 1996; Bale and Jones, 1997; Davies, 1999; Dealey, 1999).

Specific patient preparation required

⌘ If analgesia is required, allow time for this to become effective before starting the dressing

⌘ Clear enough space around the bed area to be able to carry out the procedure unhindered, removing items such as flower vases and used urinals

⌘ If available, the use of a treatment room may help in reducing the risk of cross-infection (Jamieson et al, 2002)

⌘ Allow at least 30 minutes after ward cleaning and bed making has finished before undertaking a wound dressing to reduce airborne particles. For the same reason, turn off fans, shut windows and keep activity to a minimum in the immediate vicinity during the procedure (Xavier, 1999; Nicol et al, 2000; Workman and Bennett, 2003).

During the procedure

⌘ Clean the trolley according to local policy. This may include washing the trolley with warm water and detergent and drying at the beginning of the day (Workman and Bennett, 2003)

⌘ An alcohol wipe may be used on the top of the trolley. Locally this may be done before every dressing (Jamieson et al, 2002), although unless the trolley top is visibly soiled there is no proven need (Thompson and Bullock, 1992)

⌘ Collect required equipment and place on the bottom of the trolley

⌘ Wash hands and put on clean, disposable apron

⌘ Dressing trolley is taken to the bedside

⌘ The height of the bed should be adjusted to ensure a safe working environment (Nicol et al, 2000)

⌘ The dressing pack is opened and the contents slid onto the top of the dressing trolley without contaminating the contents

⌘ Position the patient and expose the required area

⌘ Loosen the dressing covering the wound

⌘ Wash hands or use alcohol handrub
⌘ Open the inner pack touching the corners only, avoiding touching sterile inner surfaces and contents
⌘ Open any additional equipment onto the sterile field, ensuring no contamination.

If using sterile gloves

⌘ Place one hand inside disposal bag, using it as a glove in order to arrange the equipment on the sterile field. Implements such as swabs and forceps should be placed towards the edge of the sterile field near to the nurse to prevent having to reach over the sterile field (Workman and Bennett, 2003)
⌘ With hand still in the bag, hold the soiled dressing and remove, turning the bag inside out. Attach the bag to the side of the trolley nearest to the patient, to avoid taking soiled materials across the sterile field
⌘ Wash hands or use alcohol rub
⌘ If cleansing the wound, pour lotion into a gallipot, ensuring the sterile field remains dry
⌘ Put on sterile gloves.

If using forceps

⌘ Attach the disposal bag to the side of the trolley (as per glove section above)
⌘ Use one pair of forceps to arrange the contents of the dressing pack on the sterile field
⌘ Remove the soiled dressing and dispose of this, together with the forceps, into the disposal bag
⌘ If cleansing the wound, pour lotion into a gallipot, ensuring the sterile field remains dry
⌘ Wash hands or use alcohol handrub and pick up the second pair of forceps.

For both methods

⌘ The sterile drape should be placed beside the wound
⌘ Note the condition of the wound and surrounding skin to identify any wound progress or problems
⌘ Carry out wound cleansing/irrigation as required
⌘ Wound swabs of cotton wool or gauze are not advised for use on the actual wound as fibres from the material can be left on the wound (Thomas, 1993; Briggs et al, 1996; Bale and Jones, 1997)
⌘ If the surrounding area around the wound needs cleaning, this can be done with gauze dipped in cleansing solution (using each swab once)
⌘ Use fresh gauze swabs to dry around the wound
⌘ If any sharp instrument (e.g. stitch cutter) has been used, this should be disposed of in the sharps bin as soon as it has been finished with
⌘ Apply a new primary dressing and secondary dressing if required
⌘ Secure the dressing with tape or other chosen method
⌘ Throughout the procedure observe the patient's condition and reaction to the procedure
⌘ If a second nurse is available during this procedure, he/she would be able to open sterile packs and provide support for the patient.

Post-procedure

⌘ Return the bed height to a safe level

⌘ All used disposable items should be wrapped in the sterile field and placed in the disposal bag, which will then be put in the clinical waste

⌘ Remove apron and wash hands

⌘ The trolley should be cleaned as per local policy

⌘ The sharps bin and any unopened equipment should also be returned

⌘ The patient should be observed for any after effects, which should be reported

⌘ The status of the wound should be documented.

Student skill laboratory activity

⌘ Practise preparing a trolley to undertake an aseptic dressing change

⌘ Perform a simple dressing change using the aseptic technique on a manikin

⌘ Dispose of used equipment according to local policy.

Care after death/last offices

This procedure is performed after the death of a patient. It is sometimes referred to as 'laying out'. Last offices is the final procedure for a deceased patient before the body is transferred to the mortuary. During this procedure it is important to respect the values, beliefs and customs of the deceased patient.

Reasons for the procedure

⌘ To ensure that the deceased patient's dignity and respect are maintained

⌘ To facilitate a safe transfer of the deceased patient to the mortuary

⌘ To observe the deceased patient's values, belief and customs

⌘ To provide comfort to the deceased patient's family, loved ones and friends.

Pre-procedure

Equipment required

⌘ Apron

⌘ Bowl of water

⌘ Soap

- ⌘ Towels
- ⌘ Gloves
- ⌘ Clean sheets
- ⌘ Cadaver (body) bag if necessary
- ⌘ Linen skip
- ⌘ Property book
- ⌘ Identification wristbands
- ⌘ Notification of death form
- ⌘ Shroud and/or deceased patient's own clothing
- ⌘ Razor
- ⌘ Oral care equipment (toothpaste, toothbrush, mouth swabs)
- ⌘ Tape
- ⌘ Comb/brush
- ⌘ Absorbent pads
- ⌘ Spigot.

Patient preparation

- ⌘ Verify the death and ensure that this is documented in the deceased patient's nursing notes; this is usually undertaken by a doctor, but clarify with your own local policy/procedure as in some circumstances nurses can also verify a death. Specifically note the date and time when writing the entry
- ⌘ Inform the next of kin as soon as possible and establish the involvement that they may want in the last offices procedure
- ⌘ It is essential that the nurse is culturally sensitive to patients' needs and refers to relevant members of their religious faith (*Box 10.1*)
- ⌘ Some of the religious faiths will have specific aspects that need to be observed before the procedure of last offices (*Box 10.2*).

Box 10.1: Contact persons for religious faiths

Religious faith	Contact person
Buddhism	Monk or nun
Christian	Pastor/priest/vicar
Hinduism	Hindu priest (pandit)
Islam	Imam
Judaism	Rabbi or Jewish chaplain
Rastafarianism	An elder
Sikhism	Granthi (local priest)

Box 10.2: Cultural considerations after death

Buddhism	There is no single ritual to apply; however, in some traditions the body can remain at the place of death for 7 days to allow rebirth to occur. However, this may not be possible in the healthcare setting (Northcott, 2002)
Christian	Prayers and singing may be offered on death by family and relatives. The nurse usually closes the eyes and mouth and straightens the limbs — this applies to Anglicans and groups of the 'free church'
Catholics	Up to 3 hours after death, unction, a ceremony that symbolizes forgiveness, healing and reconciliation, can be given by a priest (Green, 1992)
Chinese	The family wash the body an uneven number of times in a special water that is thought to be protected by a guardian spirit; this ceremony is referred to as 'buying the spirit'. Incense may be burnt to keep evil spirits away. The body is covered in wadding and then dressed by the family in a garment that has no buttons or zips. Men will have a headdress similar to that of a Buddhist priest, while women have their hair piled high with a seven-cornered 'lotus flower hat', usually coloured gold or jade. Men may have a jade snuff bottle placed with them. Socks and shoes are placed on the feet and they in turn are bound. The Chinese may have a more eclectic approach, embracing faiths of Buddhism and Christianity (Neuberger, 1999)
Orthodox	Some older people who have visited the holy land tend to have a special shroud that they would like to wear. It is important that the orthodox priest is called for communion
Hinduism	No jewellery or religious object on the deceased should be removed. Clarify if a non-Hindu person is allowed to touch the body. Close relatives of the same sex may wish to prepare the body, including washing of the body in the practice setting. Eyes are closed and legs are straightened. Avoid cutting of hair or beard or shaving without permission. A clay lamp may be lighted or an incense stick burned (Jootun, 2002)
Islam	Close the eyes and mouth and straighten the body and limbs. The head should be turned towards the right shoulder, in doing so the body is facing towards Mecca. Avoid trimming of beard; generally, washing of the body is not undertaken in the hospital setting (Akhtar, 2002). If it is necessary for a non-Muslim to touch the body, he/she should wear gloves (Neuberger, 1999)
Judaism	People stay around the body for 8 minutes while a feather is placed over the nose and mouth to check if breathing has completely ceased (Neuberger, 1999). The son or nearest relative closes the eyes and mouth with strapping if necessary. External attachments and medical equipment can be removed if appropriate and incisions dressed. The body should be laid flat, with hands open, arms parallel and close to the body, and the legs stretched out and straightened. Bracelets and identification should be left *in situ* (Collins, 2002).

Box 10.2 *continued*: Cultural considerations after death

Judaism *continued*	Nurses should not lay the body out unless the family have indicated their express permission. The body is traditionally placed on the floor with its feet towards the door, covered with a sheet with a candle beside it. The body is not left alone, but rather watched over. In the healthcare setting, if possible, the body should be transferred to a side room where it can remain until the sexton removes it (Neuberger, 1999)
Rastafarianism	Arms placed at the side. No specific requirements other than to adhere to wishes of the deceased and family (Baxter, 2002)
Sikhism	The most important aspect of care the nurse should acknowledge are the symbols of faith, which are: — *Kesh*. Uncut hair for both men and women (nurses must not cut or trim hair, including a beard or moustache) — *Kangha*. A small wooden comb — *Kara*. A steel bangle worn on the right wrist should remain on the deceased — *Kirpan*. A short sword or dagger, although nurses can find this alarming, should also be kept on the deceased, often being worn in the form of a body belt — *Kaccha*. Unisex underwear should also remain on the deceased

From Neuberger (1999), Kaur Gill (2002)

During the procedure

- ⌘ Two staff should be working together when caring for the dead
- ⌘ Put on gloves
- ⌘ Undress the deceased patient
- ⌘ Establish if a postmortem is likely; if so, all invasive lines (for example, catheters, cannulaes, drains and nasogastric tubes) should be kept *in situ* and capped
- ⌘ The bladder may have to be manually expressed to excrete the urine after death, collect this in a bowl and dispose of as usual. In anticipation of the potential for body leakages, it may be appropriate to cover exuding wounds or pack leaking orifices
- ⌘ If appropriate to the patient's culture, wash the deceased
- ⌘ Roll the deceased to place a clean sheet underneath the patient (a sigh may be heard as air is forced out by the lungs)
- ⌘ Dress the deceased in appropriate clothing, such as a shroud or nightwear depending on his/her or family wishes and/or local policy and protocol
- ⌘ Only remove jewellery after permission from relatives; if jewellery is left *in situ*, this should be documented

⌘ All the belongings of the deceased should be checked and recorded in a property book by two members of staff and packed neatly into an appropriate bag

⌘ To ensure correct identification for mortuary staff, an identification band is placed on a wrist and one ankle (usually one on either side of the body if possible). This should include the name, hospital number, date of birth, date of death and ward/unit. A notification of death form should be completed and applied usually to the front of the clothing that the deceased is dressed in. The body is then wrapped in a clean sheet and secured with tape to ensure safe and dignified transfer

⌘ If the body is identified as being 'high risk' or leaking excessive bodily fluid, then a cadaver (body) bag may be required

⌘ Depending on local policy or protocol, a notification of death form may be placed on top of the wrapped body; then the body should be covered with a clean, loose sheet (Nearney, 1998a,b,c; Docherty, 2000; Nicol et al, 2000)

⌘ Arrange for the transfer of the body.

Post-procedure

⌘ Remove and dispose of equipment as necessary

⌘ Support and comfort relatives, providing them with contact details of appropriate people and procedures to follow

⌘ Contact any other relevant people

⌘ Support inpatients in the surrounding area who may have known the deceased

⌘ Staff may require time to debrief.

Student skill laboratory activity

⌘ The facilitator should be aware that this procedure may cause a number of emotions in students, and this should be addressed accordingly

⌘ Assemble the equipment required to 'lay out' a body

⌘ Practise 'laying out' a manikin.

Ear irrigation

Ear irrigation to remove wax or cerumen is one of the most common procedures carried out by nurses and doctors. It is an invasive procedure and involves a pulsed-water jet system using a narrow tube connected to a pump to remove wax from the external auditory meatus.

Reasons for the procedure

⌘ To remove obstruction of the external auditory meatus caused by excess cerumen. This is a common problem (Kamien, 1999) that affects all ages, and can cause the client a number of symptoms — discomfort, irritation, pain, vertigo or tinnitus

⌘ To remove foreign bodies that are not hydroscopic, for example peas as these swell under the influence of fluid.

Pre-procedure

Equipment required

⌘ Pulsed-water jet system in working order

⌘ Waterproof sheet — to drape across patient's shoulder and chest

⌘ Absorbent towel to cover waterproof sheet

⌘ Auriscope with a range of speculums

⌘ Headlight — to ensure direct vision of the ear and external auditory meatus

⌘ Jug containing tap water warmed to 37°C

⌘ Kidney dish or Noots tank to receive water as it exits the ear

⌘ Jobson probe with cotton wool to clean and dry external auditory meatus.

Specific patient preparation required

⌘ Ensure that no contraindications exists, such as a perforation (past or present) of the tympanic membrane, the presence of a grommet, ear infection, uncooperative young children and some older clients who have dementia

⌘ Before commencing the procedure, both ears should be examined externally (pre-aural and post-aural) and internally to observe for abnormalities such as previous surgery scars, trauma, signs of infection and extent of cerumenous discharge to be removed

⌘ The external auditory meatus is S-shaped, and to gain good visualization this needs straightening

⌘ The client is asked to sit in a well-supported, comfortable, upright position to reduce the risk of movement during the procedure, which could result in movement of the irrigator tip and therefore possible trauma to the client

⌘ This procedure may be uncomfortable but it should not be painful; any pain the client experiences must be reported to the nurse immediately. In this case the procedure should be stopped and the ear inspected to eliminate any trauma. Sharp et al (1990) and Price (1997) have identified that although ear irrigation is a common procedure it is also invasive and has the potential to cause discomfort or trauma

⌘ The nurse must ensure that the client is protected from any resultant water leakage by placing the waterproof sheet and holding the Noots tank/kidney dish under the pinna as this can help the patient feel involved in the treatment.

During the procedure

⌘ Fill the irrigator system with water following manufacturer's instructions

⌘ The tap water used should be at 37°C — if it is too hot or cold it can stimulate the semicircular canals, which will result in the client feeling dizzy (Harkin and Vaz, 2003) and may cause a nystagmus (involuntary flickering movements of the eyeball)

⌘ Switch on the equipment to circulate the water through the system and to eliminate any trapped air and/or cold water. The initial flow of water is discarded and the patient becomes familiar with the noise. The patient can be reassured by allowing him/her to feel the flow of the water on the fingers before ear irrigation starts

⌘ Under direct vision, with the use of a headlight to illuminate the ear and external auditory meatus, place the angle tip of the irrigator in the base of the external meatus a short way (using the intertragal notch as an entry point) and aim upwards and slightly backwards so that the jet of water travels along the roof of the external auditory meatus and then falls behind the obstruction, causing it to move towards the pinna and therefore be expelled

⌘ If the patient has a perforation of the tympanic membrane, this may cause them to suddenly swallow. If this happens the irrigation must be stopped and the cause investigated as water entering the middle ear may cause a middle-ear infection (Stubbs, 2000)

⌘ The external auditory meatus must be checked at frequent intervals to examine the effectiveness of the treatment and to ensure that any trauma is identified and, if necessary, the treatment discontinued. Once the tympanic membrane can be visualized, the irrigation must be stopped

⌘ With the aid of the headlight, the ear should be dried under direct vision using a Jobson probe with cotton wool to reduce the risk of discomfort and infection.

Post-procedure

⌘ Any abrasions to the external auditory meatus predisposes it to otitis externa and static water can contain *Pseudomonas aeruginosa* (Campos et al, 1998). Common complications following ear syringing are otitis externa, pain and external auditory meatus trauma (Bapat et al, 2001)

⌘ Complete patient documentation

⌘ Patient education — the nurse must discuss with the client the natural cleaning process of his/her ears, as the ear is a self-cleaning organ with both the dead cells of the epidermis and cerumen migrating out of the external auditory meatus. Sharp et al (1990) identified that if clients understand the natural cleaning properties of the ear and external auditory meatus, they are less likely to feel the need to keep their ears 'wax free'

⌘ The client should be discouraged from using tools such as cotton buds or hair grips, as these may remove some cerumen but will push other cerumen further along the external auditory meatus towards the tympanic membrane, where it can harden and require ear irrigation to remove it.

Wound swab

Swabbing a wound involves using a sterile cotton-tipped swab to sample the exudate from the surface of a wound.

Reasons for the procedure

- ⌘ To identify harmful organisms within a wound
- ⌘ To facilitate the process of diagnosis
- ⌘ To prescribe correct antibiotics
- ⌘ To inform dressing choice.

Pre-procedure

Equipment required

- ⌘ Dressing trolley
- ⌘ Wound pack containing gauze swabs, plastic pots and sterile towel
- ⌘ Appropriate dressing(s) and materials for securing the dressing
- ⌘ Clinical waste bag
- ⌘ Sachets of normal saline
- ⌘ Pre-labelled sterile wound swab
- ⌘ Microbiology request form
- ⌘ Gloves x 2
- ⌘ Apron.

Specific patient preparation required

- ⌘ Position the patient, exposing the wound site
- ⌘ Offer analgesics as necessary
- ⌘ Loosen existing dressing(s).

During the procedure

- ⌘ Wash hands and put on apron
- ⌘ Set out equipment on a trolley and take to the patient
- ⌘ Prepare sterile field
- ⌘ Put on gloves, remove dressings and discard into a clinical waste bag
- ⌘ Remove gloves, wash hands and re-glove

⌘ Identify the area that the wound swab is going to be taken from. It should be taken from an area of viable tissue where there are clinical signs of infection. Avoid swabbing collections of pus, eschar tissue or yellow fibrous slough (Cuzzell, 1993; Kiernan, 1998), as the latter will not indicate the cause of infection but rather dead organisms and debris. In large wounds the whole wound surface should be swabbed

⌘ Separate the cotton-tipped swab from the container by twisting clockwise and removing it with your dominant hand. Avoid contaminating the swab

⌘ In the other hand, retain the plastic cover ready to receive the swab

⌘ Hold the swab between finger and thumb and use a rotating action to take a sample from all areas of the wound using a zig-zag motion (Donovan, 1998; Lawrence, 1999)

⌘ Replace the swab in the plastic cover

⌘ Redress the wound with an appropriate dressing.

Post-procedure

⌘ Reposition patient

⌘ Date and time the wound swab label and microbiology form

⌘ Send swab to laboratory according to local policy.

Student skill laboratory activity

⌘ Identify the equipment required to undertake a wound swab

⌘ Practise taking a wound swab on a manikin.

References

Akhtar S (2002) Nursing with dignity. Part 8: Islam. *Nurs Times* **98**(16): 40–2

Bale S, Jones V (1997) *Wound Care Nursing. A Patient-centred Approach*. Bailliere Tindall, London

Bapat U, Nia J, Bance M (2001) Severe audiovestibular loss following ear syringing for wax removal. *J Laryngol Otol* **115**(5): 410–11

Baxter C (2002) Nursing with dignity. Part 5: Rastafarianism. *Nurs Times* **98**(13): 42–3

Briggs M, Wilson S, Fuller A (1996) The principles of aseptic technique in wound care. *Prof Nurse* **11:** 805–10

Campos A, Arias A, Betancor L et al (1998) Influence of human wet cerumen on the growth of common and pathogenic bacteria of the ear. *J Laryngol Otol* **112:** 613–16

Collier M (1996) Trauma injury nursing in A&E. *Nurs Times* **92**(20): 74–9

Collins A (2002) Nursing with dignity. Part 1: Judaism. *Nurs Times* **98**(9): 34–5

Cuzzell JZ (1993) The right way to culture a wound. *Am J Nurs* **93**(5): 48–50

Davies C (1999) Cleansing rites and wrongs. *Nurs Times* **95**(43): 71–3

Dealey C (1999) *The Care of Wounds. A Guide for Nurses.* 2nd edn. Blackwell Science, Oxford

Docherty B (2000) Care of the dying patient. *Prof Nurse* **15:** 752

Donovan S (1998) Wound infection and wound swabbing. *Prof Nurse* **13:** 757–9

Green J (1992) Christianity. *Nurs Times* **88**(3): 26–9

Harkin H, Vaz F (2003) Nursing patients with common problems of the ear and hearing. In: Brooker C, Nicol M, eds. *Nursing Adults: The Practice of Caring.* Mosby, Edinburgh

Jamieson EM, McCall JM, Whyte LA (2002) *Clinical Nursing Practice.* 4th edn. Churchill Livingstone, Edinburgh

Jootun D (2002) Nursing with dignity. Part 7: Hinduism. *Nurs Times* **98**(15): 38–40

Kamien M (1999) Which cerumenolytic? *Aust Family Phys* **28**(8): 817–28

Kaur Gill B (2002) Nursing with dignity. Part 6: Sikhism. *Nurs Times* **98**(14): 39–41

Kiernan M (1998) Role of swabbing in wound infection management. *Community Nurse* **4**(6): 45–6

Lawrence J (1999) Swab taking. *J Wound Care* **8:** 251

Myers J (1982) Modern plastic surgical dressings. *Health Soc Serv J* **92:** 336–7

Nearney L (1998a) Last offices — 1. *Nurs Times* **94**(26): suppl 1–2

Nearney L (1998b) Last offices — 2. *Nurs Times* **94**(27): suppl 1–2

Nearney L (1998c) Last offices — 3. *Nurs Times* **94**(28): suppl 3–4

Neuberger J (1999) *Dying Well: A Guide to Enabling a Good Death.* Hochland and Hochland, Hale

Nicol M, Bavin C, Bedford-Turner S, Cronin P, Rawlings-Anderson K (2000) *Essential Nursing Skills.* Mosby, Edinburgh

Northcott N (2002) Nursing with dignity. Part 2: Buddhism. *Nurs Times* **98**(10): 36–8m

Price J (1997) Problems of ear syringing. *Practice Nurse* **114**(2): 26–8

Sharp JF, Wilson JA, Ross L, Barr-Hamilton RM (1990) Ear wax removal. A survey of current practice. *Br Med J* **301:** 1251–3

Stubbs G (2000) Ear-syringing and aural care. *Nurs Times* **96**(42): 35

Thomas S (1993) Comparing non-woven filmated and woven gauze swabs. *J Wound Care* **2**(1): 35–41

Thompson G, Bullock D (1992) To clean or not to clean? *Nurs Times* **88**(34): 66–8

Workman BA, Bennett CL (2003) *Key Nursing Skills.* Whurr Publishers, London

Xavier G (1999) Asepsis. *Nurs Stand* **13**(36): 49–53

Further reading

Beldon P (2001) Recognising wound infection. *Nurs Times* **97**(3): 251

Blunt J (2001) Wound cleansing: ritualistic or research-based practice? *Nurs Stand* **16**(1): 33–6

Bree-Williams FJ, Waterman H (1996) An examination of nurses' practice when performing aseptic technique for wound dressings. *J Adv Nurs* **23:** 48–54

Bridson EY (1990) *The Oxford Manual.* 6th edn. Unipath, Basingstoke

Casey G (2003) Nutritional support in wound healing. *Nurs Stand* **16**(1): 33–6

Castille K (1998) Suturing. *Nurs Stand* **12**(41): 41–8

Clark A (2004) Understanding the principles of suturing a minor skin lesion. *Nurs Times* **100**(29): 32–4

Clark JE (1990) *Clinical Nursing Manual*. Prentice Hall, London

Collier M (2003) The elements of wound assessment. *Nurs Times* **99**(13): 48–9

Coopey S (2001) Ear syringing: a case for clinical governace. *J Community Nurs* **15**(1): 20–2

Cutting KF (1997) Wounds and evidence of infection. *Nurs Stand* **11**(25): 49–52

Cutting K, Harding K (1994) Criteria for identifying wound infection. *J Wound Care* **3:** 198–201

Davies C (1999) Cleansing rites and wrongs. *Nurs Times* **95**(43): 71–5

Dearden C, Donnell J, Donnelly J, Dunlop M (2001) Traumatic wounds: cleansing and dressing. *Nurs Times* **97**(28): 50–2

Department of Health (2001) *Reforming Emergency Care*. DoH, London

Dimond B (2002) *Legal Aspects of Law*. 3rd edn. Longman, Harlow

Flanagan M (1997) *Wound Management*. Churchill Livingstone, Edinburgh

Gilchrist B (1996) Wound infection. *J Wound Care* **5:** 386–92

Gould D (1999) *Wound Management*. Nursing Times Books, London

Harker J (2002) Promoting best practice in leg ulcer assessment. *Nurs Times* **98**(44): 60–1

Harkin H (2000) Evidence based ear care. *Primary Health Care* **10**(81): 25–30

Hines J (1997) Making the right noises: caring for hearing impaired patients. *Nurs Times* **93**(31): 33

Jones I, Molton C (1998) Use of an electric ear syringe in the emergency department. *J Accid Emerg Med* **15**(5): 327–8

Kingsley A, Winfield-Davies S (2003) Audit of wound swab sampling: why protocols could improve practice. *Prof Nurse* **18:** 338–43

Lawton S, Rich A (1999) Reaction stations. *Nurs Times* **95**(37): 10–11

Lippert H (1999) *Compendium: Wounds and Wound Management*. Hartmann, Heidenheim

Memel D, Langley C, Watkins C, Laue B, Birchall M, Bachmann M (2002) Effectiveness of ear syringing in general practice: a randomised controlled trial and patients' experiences. *Br J Gen Pract* **52**(484): 906–11

Moorehead RJ, Whiteside MC (1999) *Wound Management: Theory and Practice*. Nursing Times Books, London

Nursing and Midwifery Council (2002) *Code of Professional Conduct*. NMC, London

Nursing and Midwifery Council (2002) *Guidelines for Records and Record Keeping*. NMC, London

Peters J (1999) Saving face. *Nurs Times* **95**(Suppl 37): 8–9

Purcell D (2003) *Minor Injuries: A Clinical Guide for Nurses*. Churchill Livingstone, London

Royal College of Nursing (1998) *Clinical Practice Guidelines*. RCN Institute, Manchester

Starr S, MacLeod T (2003) Wound swabbing technique. *Nurs Times* **99**(5): 57–9

Thurgood K, Thurgood G (1995) Ear syringing: a clinical skill. *Br J Nurs* **4:** 682–7

Thwaites C, Farrar J (2003) Preventing and treating tetanus. *BMJ* **326:** 117–18

Tomlinson D (1987) To clean or not to clean? *Nurs Times* **87**(37): 71–5

Trengove NJ, Stacey MC, McGechie DF, Mata S (1996) Qualitative bacteriology and leg ulcer healing. *J Wound Care* **5:** 277–80

Vickerstaff E (2001) Safe syringing. *Practice Nurse* **21**(7): 24–8

Walsh M, Kent A (2001) *Accident and Emergency Nursing*. 4th edn. Butterworth Heinemann, Oxford

Wardrope J, Edhouse J (2000) *The Management of Wounds and Burns*. Oxford University Press, Oxford

Index

Notes